Lecture Notes of the Institute for Computer Sciences, Social Informatics and Telecommunications Engineering 456

The LNICST series publishes ICST's conferences, symposia and workshops. It reports state-of-the-art results in areas related to the scope of the Institute.

LNICST reports state-of-the-art results in areas related to the scope of the Institute. The type of material published includes

- Proceedings (published in time for the respective event)
- Other edited monographs (such as project reports or invited volumes)

LNICST topics span the following areas:

- General Computer Science
- E-Economy
- E-Medicine
- Knowledge Management
- Multimedia
- Operations, Management and Policy
- Social Informatics
- Systems

Susanna Spinsante · Grazia Iadarola ·
Alessia Paglialonga · Federico Tramarin
Editors

IoT Technologies
for HealthCare

9th EAI International Conference, HealthyIoT 2022
Braga, Portugal, November 16–18, 2022
Proceedings

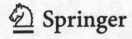
Springer

Editors
Susanna Spinsante ⓘ
Università Politecnica delle Marche
Ancona, Italy

Grazia Iadarola ⓘ
Università Politecnica delle Marche
Ancona, Italy

Alessia Paglialonga ⓘ
CNR-Istituto di Elettronica e di Ingegneria
dell'Informazione e delle Telecomunicazioni
Milan, Italy

Federico Tramarin ⓘ
Università di Modena e Reggio Emilia
Modena, Italy

ISSN 1867-8211 ISSN 1867-822X (electronic)
Lecture Notes of the Institute for Computer Sciences, Social Informatics
and Telecommunications Engineering
ISBN 978-3-031-28662-9 ISBN 978-3-031-28663-6 (eBook)
https://doi.org/10.1007/978-3-031-28663-6

This Springer imprint is published by the registered company Springer Nature Switzerland AG
The registered company address is: Gewerbestrasse 11, 6330 Cham, Switzerland

Preface

We are delighted to introduce the proceedings of the ninth edition of the 2022 European Alliance for Innovation (EAI) International Conference on IoT Technologies for Health-Care (HealthyIoT). Traditionally, this conference covers multiple aspects of using IoT in healthcare and brings together technology experts, researchers, industry experts and international authorities contributing towards the design, development, and deployment of healthcare solutions based on IoT technologies, standards, and procedures. This year the emphasis was on using IoT in healthcare for societal benefit – towards improved health and wellbeing for everyone.

The technical program of HealthyIoT 2022 consisted of 11 full papers, in oral presentation sessions at the conference, and 2 invited papers. The oral sessions included high-quality technical presentations of the papers submitted to the HealthyIoT 2022 tracks, i.e. a Main Track, and an Invited Track. Accepted papers were presented in two sessions, namely "Analysis of Measurement Data in IoT Technologies for Health", and "IoT Applications in Research and Clinical Practice".

Coordination with the steering chairs, Imrich Chlamtac, Ivan Miguel Serrano Pires and Aleksandar Jevremovic, was essential for the success of the conference. We sincerely appreciate their constant support and guidance. It was also a great pleasure to work with such an excellent organizing committee team for their hard work in organizing and supporting the conference. In particular, the Technical Program Committee, led by our TPC Co-Chairs, Grazia Iadarola, Alessia Paglialonga and Federico Tramarin, who coordinated and contributed to the peer-review process of technical papers, and made a high-quality technical program. We are also grateful to the Conference Manager, Kristina Havlickova, for her support, and to all the authors who submitted their papers to the HealthyIoT 2022 conference, sharing their knowledge, experience, and genuine enthusiasm.

We strongly believe that the HealthyIoT conference provides a good forum for all researcher, developers, and practitioners to discuss scientific and technical aspects that are relevant to IoT technologies for healthcare. We also expect that future HealthyIoT conferences will be as successful and stimulating, as indicated by the contributions presented in this volume.

Susanna Spinsante
Grazia Iadarola
Alessia Paglialonga
Federico Tramarin

Conference Organization

Steering Committee

Imrich Chlamtac   Bruno Kessler Professor, University of Trento, Italy

Susanna Spinsante   Università Politecnica delle Marche, Italy

Ivan Miguel Serrano Pires   Instituto Politécnico de Viseu, Portugal

Aleksandar Jevremovic   Singidunum University, Serbia

Organizing Committee

General Chair

Susanna Spinsante   Università Politecnica delle Marche, Italy

General Co-chair

Aleksandar Jevremovic   Singidunum University, Serbia

TPC Co-chairs

Alessia Paglialonga   Istituto di Elettronica e di Ingegneria dell'Informazione e delle Telecomunicazioni (IEIIT), National Research Council (CNR) of Italy

Grazia Iadarola   Università Politecnica delle Marche, Italy

Federico Tramarin   Università di Modena e Reggio Emilia, Italy

Sponsorship and Exhibit Chair

Nuno M. Garcia   Universidade da Beira Interior, Portugal

Local Chair

Bruno Silva   Universidade da Beira Interior, Portugal

Workshops Chair

Bruno Silva   Universidade da Beira Interior, Portugal

Publicity and Social Media Chair

Nuno Cruz Garcia   Universidade de Lisboa, Portugal

Publications Chair

Ivan Miguel Serrano Pires   Instituto Politécnico de Viseu, Portugal

Web Chair

Gonçalo Marques   Polytechnic of Coimbra, Portugal

Technical Program Committee

Alvaro Hernandez	University of Alcalá, Spain
Antonio Ramón Jiménez Ruiz	Spanish Council for Scientific Research, Spain
Ciprian Dobre	University Politehnica of Bucharest, Romania
Dušanka Bošković	University of Sarajevo, Bosnia and Herzegovina
Emmanuel Conchon	University of Limoges, France
Ennio Gambi	Università Politecnica delle Marche, Italy
Francesco Lamonaca	University of Calabria, Italy
Fernando Ribeiro	University of Minho, Portugal
Hugo Daniel Peixoto	University of Minho, Portugal
Ivan Ganchev	University of Limerick, Ireland University of Plovdiv "Paisii Hilendarski", Bulgaria
John Gialelis	University of Patras, Greece
José Alberto Benítez-Andrades	University of León, Spain
Karim Keshavjee	University of Toronto, Canada
Lidia Bajenaru	National Institute for Research and Development in Informatics – ICI Bucharest, Romania
Maji Soumyajyoti	Harvard University, USA
Manuela Montangero	University of Modena and Reggio Emilia, Italy
Marco Sarac	Singidunum University, Serbia
Rossitza Ivanova Goleva	New Bulgarian University, Bulgaria

Saeed Mian Qaisar	Effat University, Jeddah, Saudi Arabia
Sandeep Pirbhulal	Norwegian University of Science and Technology, Norway
Vladimir Trajkovik	SS. Cyril and Methodius University in Skopje, Republic of North Macedonia

Contents

Analysis of Measurement Data in IoT Technologies for Health

Automatic Wardrobe for Blind People

Luís Silva[1], Daniel Rocha[2,3], Vítor Carvalho[2,3(✉)], João Sena Esteves[2],
and Filomena Soares[2]

[1] School of Engineering, University of Minho, Campus of Azurém, Guimarães, Portugal
a84100@alunos.uminho.pt

[2] Centro Algoritmi, University of Minho, Campus of Azurém, Guimarães, Portugal
id8057@alunos.uminho.pt, vcarvalho@ipca.pt, {sena,
fsoares}@dei.uminho.pt

[3] 2Ai, School of Technology, Campus of IPCA, Barcelos, Portugal

Abstract. In the last years, the integration of handicapped individuals in society has gained significant attention and is being strongly stimulated by several activities. In this context, technology has major importance. Several technological solutions that help handicapped people in their daily routine, allowing their integration into society, have emerged. However, besides all efforts that have been made, still exist some challenges related to specific basic tasks in blind people's daily routines. Namely, the management and identification of personal garments could become a complex and time-consuming task. For this specific task, these people depend on their relatives for choosing the exact clothes desired. In this way, and based on the problems presented, this paper proposes the development of an automatic wardrobe capable to assist blind people. This proposal is integrated in a work under development of a prototype of a mechatronic system for the choice and management of garments. The proposed solution seeks to provide an improvement in the quality of life of blind people.

Keywords: Blind People · Automatic Wardrobe · Garments

1 Introduction

Over the last years, there has been an effort to develop technologies that provide handicapped people access to information and knowledge. In the specific case of blind people, there are plenty of technological solutions that help in activities of daily routine. However, there are several challenges related to daily basic tasks, especially in the choice of personal garments. These individuals cannot choose autonomously the desired clothing and, consequently, the identification of features on clothing becomes a slow and difficult task. This paper presents an automatic wardrobe that allows an improvement in the quality of life and well-being of blind people. The main goal of the work under development is the design, development, and validation in ACAPO (Portuguese Association of Blind and Amblyope People) of a prototype of a mechatronic system for the choice and management of garments that includes the automatic wardrobe. In the future, this

© ICST Institute for Computer Sciences, Social Informatics and Telecommunications Engineering 2023
Published by Springer Nature Switzerland AG 2023. All Rights Reserved
S. Spinsante et al. (Eds.): HealthyIoT 2022, LNICST 456, pp. 3–13, 2023.
https://doi.org/10.1007/978-3-031-28663-6_1

physical system will be integrated with a mobile application for iOS that is part of the system MyEyes [1–3] and will allow a virtual wardrobe replication in the smartphone, making management easier and intuitive.

This paper has seven sections. After the introduction given in Sect. 1, Sect. 2 describes the state of the art; Sect. 3 presents the system overview; the hardware architecture and the software architecture are presented in Sect. 4 and Sect. 5, respectively; the preliminary results are presented in Sect. 6; Sect. 7 presents the conclusions and some ideas regarding future work.

2 Previous Work

The literature review shows that there are several solutions to help people in the choice of personal garments. These solutions are based on virtual wardrobes, a concept with a great increase in the last years. It is important to know the consumer's attitudes about this new approach. In [4], Perry et al. present a study that focuses on consumers' acceptance of smart virtual wardrobes. The results show that there is a great acceptance of the concept of smart wardrobes. The utility and ease of use are key factors for the choice.

A survey carried out encompassing all the delegations of ACAPO (Portuguese Association of Blind and Amblyope People) allowed the identification of several problems regarding garments identification by blind people [5]. The main goal of the survey was to recognize both the importance of garment identification and several technological solutions existing for this specific community. It was possible to identify that there are several solutions, but they do not focus on the aesthetic aspect of managing garments. *MyEyes,* presented in [1–3] was developed to overcome this gap. The solution is based on a system that integrates a mobile application with an Arduino board allowing users to have a virtual wardrobe with their garments. Near Field Communication (NFC) tags attached to the garments allow the addition of clothing items to the virtual wardrobe. A general overview of a possible prototype implementation for this solution was presented in [6].

In [7] is presented a solution to help blind people match garments. The system integrates NFC technology with a smartphone, allowing visually impaired people to choose the desired clothes. The solution presented in [8] explores NFC technology combined with Quick Response (QR) technology with the main goal of developing a clothing matching system with audio description.

Solutions whose main target is people without any or partial visual disability are in a crescent rising with more implementations emerging. Goh et al. [9] propose a system that integrates tags with Radio Frequency Identification (RFID) technology, allowing unique identification of clothing items. The system is based on RFID tag reading and the user obtains the features data that were saved on each tag. This system is controlled by an application that allows garment management and suggests clothing items based on several criteria, such as style, color, material, and user's mood. Due to the increasing demand for implementations that aid in garments management, some fashion brands present different solutions developed to help people plan what to wear. In 2017, Amazon presented the Echo Look [10] based on a kit with a camera that allows garments photo capture and cataloguing of outfits. This method also suggests combinations based on meteorology and users' preferences. The mobile application Fashion API [11] is a closet that plans what to purchase and adds garments based on QR code reading. Another mobile application is the Smart Closet [12], which plans combinations to wear and allows the addition of clothing items based on photo capture. TailorTags [13] is a system that uses smart tags to detect garments automatically. Also suggests combinations based on users' preferences or meteorology. Table 1 summarizes the advantages and limitations of the systems previously described.

Table 1. Advantages and limitations of several smart wardrobe solutions.

Solutions	Advantages	Limitations
MyEyes [1–3]	Manage garments based on RFID tags reading	Does not implement artificial intelligence algorithms
"An IoT smart clothing system for the visually impaired using NFC technology" [7]	Manage garments based on NFC technology	Does not integrate a physical prototype
"My best shirt with the right pants: improving the outfits of visually impaired people with QR codes and NFC tags" [8]	Manage garments based on the combination of NFC and QR technology	Does not implement artificial intelligence algorithms
"Developing a smart wardrobe system" [9]	Adds clothing items to the wardrobe based on RFID tags reading	Does not implement artificial intelligence algorithms
Echo Look [10]	Suggests advice based on weather and personal trend	Photo capture at an ideal distance could be a problem
Fashion API [11]	Adds clothing items to the virtual wardrobe based on QR code reading	Only integrates a mobile application
Smart Closet [12]	Adds clothing items to the virtual wardrobe based on photo capture	Does not implement artificial intelligence algorithms
TailorTags [13]	Adds clothing items to the virtual wardrobe based on wireless tags detection	Only integrates a mobile application

Besides all efforts to develop systems to help blind people, except for solutions presented in [1–3, 7], and [8], the systems in Table 1 focus on solutions that help blind people. So, based on the gaps and limitations of the solutions presented in Table 1, an automatic wardrobe capable of improving the quality of life of blind people is presented in this paper.

3 System Overview

The developed system has two main parts: the physical prototype and the system software. The system integrates an NFC reader whose responsibility is to read the tags attached to each garment. The circular movement of garments is the responsibility of a stepper motor screwed to the wardrobe's roof. In each hanger is included a servo motor that allows a 180 degrees rotation when the photo capture takes place. This rotation allows the capture of a front and a back photo. On photo capture, on each capture moment, two photos are taken (a top and a bottom) and submitted to a stitching algorithm. This system is based on a Raspberry Pi 4, which is responsible for data processing and sending the data to the user when requested. Regarding to lightning, the wardrobe contains an inside illumination to evidence garments features and eliminate any kind of reflection with the main goal of providing a controlled system for garment photo capture allowing the avoidance of dark fields and shadows (Fig. 1).

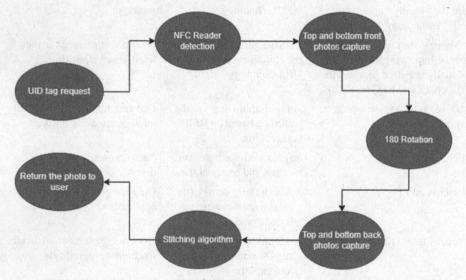

Fig. 1. System overview

4 Hardware Architecture

The system encompasses four phases: NFC reading, photo capturing, hanger rotating, and circular movement. The NFC module reads the tags attached to each garment allowing the obtainment of the UID code associated with each tag. The photo capture is the responsibility of a vision system with one camera. Due to the impossibility of capturing the full of view of a garment with only one shoot, a small servo motor is connected to the camera to rotate 180 degrees allowing two positions on photo capture. With this solution, a top photo and a bottom photo are taken and submitted to a stitching algorithm that joins the photos, originating a complete garment photo. In each hanger, there is attached a servo motor providing a 180 degrees rotation which allows the capture of a front and a back photo. Regarding the circular movement inside the wardrobe, a stepper motor was screwed to the roof whose shaft had connected to a circular platform where the servo motors attached to the hangers were connected.

4.1 Illumination

Illumination is a key factor in photo capture. The garments should be illuminated avoiding any dark fields so, the colour should be white and diffused. The type of illumination chosen was a LED strip that allows great flexibility for a low price. This strip is constituted by hundreds of LEDs that emit light with a temperature of about 6000K being located on the wall where the cameras are allowing a higher focus on each garment.

4.2 Prototype Design

The goal of the project presented in this paper is to develop an automatic wardrobe able to improve the quality of life and well-being of blind people. For this proof of concept, it was considered a small wardrobe from IKEA [14] with the following dimensions: 50x30x80 cm.

As mentioned before, on the wardrobe roof, there is a stepper motor responsible for the circular movement. A circular platform is coupled to the motor shaft that supports the weight of all servo motors attached to each hanger. The servo motors responsible for a 180 degrees rotation of each garment are attached to the circular platform inferior surface. The NFC reader is screwed to a side wall to allow the collision and detection of User Identification (UID) associated with each tag. The camera is connected to a small servo responsible for a 180 degrees rotation allowing the capture of two photos (Fig. 2).

The microcontroller used as a base for the system implementation was the Raspberry Pi 3B + board, which is used in complex projects, offering great versatility for a low price. The 40 pins on board can be used for several functions, such as Inter-Integrated Circuit (I2C), Serial Peripheral Interface (SPI), and Universal Asynchronous Receiver-Transmitter (UART) communication. This minicomputer has 1GB of RAM and has inserted a Secure Digital (SD) Card with 16GB of storage that allows the installation of the Raspbian Operative System. For the tags reading was used a PN532 module that communicates via NFC. This module allows I2C, SPI, and UART connection to the Raspberry Pi board and can detect tags up to 4 cm of distance.

Two types of actuators were used: servo motors and a stepper motor. Each servo motor was connected to the hangers to warrant a 180 degrees rotation of each garment when the photo capture takes place. A small servo was connected to the camera to allow two positions on photo capture. The stepper motor was screwed to the roof allowing garments movement inside the wardrobe. This stepper is connected to ULN2003 driver that controls the motor rotation.

For the photo capture, it was used one OV5647 camera. This module integrates the camera with a small board responsible for the connection to the BCM2835 processor via Channel State Information (CSI) communication. The camera has 5 MP and delivers images with a resolution up to 2592 x 1944. This module is connected to the Raspberry Pi over the Channel State Information (CSI) bus.

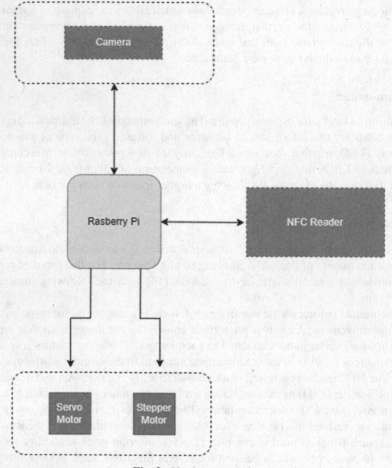

Fig. 2. Hardware overview

5 Software Architecture

A control software was developed in order to test and validate the wardrobe automatism. The state machine presented in Fig. 3 describes the functioning of the system, which has six states: READY, STEPPER, DETECTION, CAPTURE, SERVO, and STITCH. When the user requests a garment, the initial state READY is changed to STEPPER. In this state, the stepper motor that controls the garments movement inside the wardrobe is triggered and moves until the tag with the requested UID is detected and stops. The state changes to DETECTION and the UID tag is displayed. Then, the system changes its state to CAPTURE, and a top and bottom front photos of the garment are taken. The system state changes to SERVO and the servo motor is triggered, performing a 180 degrees rotation. After this rotation, the system returns to CAPTURE state, and a top and bottom back photos are taken. The system then changes to the STITCH state, where a stitching algorithm combines the photos. The stitching algorithm allows solving a problem related to the impossibility of capturing the total full of view of each garment with only one camera shoot. So, this algorithm, which is part of the OpenCV library, combines images based on keypoint detection and overlaps common points on each picture.

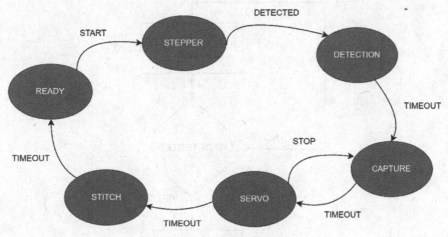

Fig. 3. System State machine

6 Preliminary Results

Some preliminary results allow the validation of the different modules previously presented. The automatisms responsible for the movement are already developed and implemented. The stepper motor has a circular platform connected to the shaft and is connected to ULN2003 which is a driver that controls the motor rotation. This is a module that integrates the motor and the driver on the same board. The circular platform is where the servo motors, responsible for each hanger, are connected. Each motor has a hanger connected to the shaft to warrant the rotation on the photo capture. The control software developed allows the test and validation of the wardrobe automatism, i.e., the integration between the hardware and the software. The flowchart presented in Fig. 4 describes the flow of the automatism implemented.

The system flow starts with the stepper motor being triggered until the tag detection. When the requested tag is detected, a top and a bottom front photos are taken, and the servo motor rotates 180 degrees in order to a top and bottom back photos be captured. Next, the photos are submitted to a stitching algorithm originating two photos (a front and a back). This stitching algorithm was implemented to solve a gap related to the garment photo full of view. As can be seen in Fig. 5, this method was capable of effectively detecting several common points in each photo and matching them in the final photo.

The developed automatic wardrobe has the main capability of guaranteeing a controlled system on photo capture avoiding dark fields and shadows. A garment was tested on the automatic wardrobe to show the accuracy of the controlled system on photo capture. Figures 6a) and 6b) show that in capture outside the controlled system is not

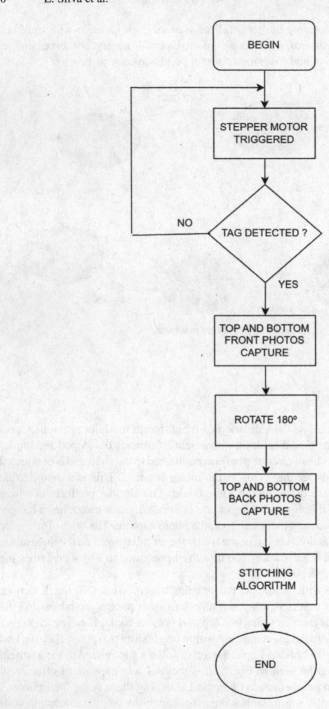

Fig. 4. System Flowchart

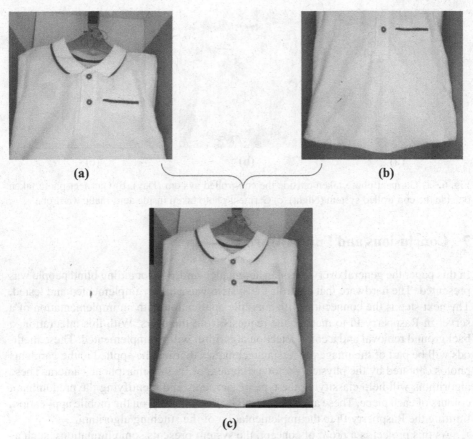

(a)   **(b)**

(c)

Fig. 5. a) Garment Top photo Algorithm Test. b) – Garment Bottom photo Algorithm Test. c) – Garment Complete Photo

guaranteed a photo without shadows or dark fields. On the contrary, inside the automatic wardrobe, the photo is taken, and the illumination evidences the garment features and eliminates any kind of reflection (Fig. 6c).

Comparing the proposed system with the solutions described in Sect. 2, only in [9] is presented a physical system. However, that system has only the capability of storing the garments, contrasting with the system proposed in this paper, that is capable of not only storing the garments but also capturing garments photos inside the physical system, as well as integrating an automatism that guarantees the pieces movement when requested by the user. The other solutions mainly focus on management apps with wireless technology. This feature is also present in the system proposed in this paper, which uses NFC communication by attaching a tag to each garment in order to ease the addition and removal of pieces.

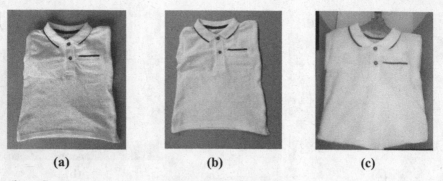

(a)   (b)   (c)

Fig. 6. a) Garment photo taken outside the con-trolled system (Day). b) Garment photo taken outside the con-trolled system (Night). c) Garment photo taken inside auto-matic wardrobe

7   Conclusions and Future Work

In this paper the general overview of an automatic wardrobe for aiding blind people was presented. The hardware that controls the system was already implemented and tested. The next step is the connection with a mobile application with an implementation of a server in Raspberry Pi to manage the requests from the users. With this integration, a background removal and a color detection algorithm will be implemented. These methods will be part of the image processing techniques that will be applied to the garments photos captured by the physical prototype camera or by the smartphone camera. These algorithms will help classifying the type of garments and identifying the predominant colours of each piece. These approaches will be implemented on the mobile application, limiting the Raspberry Pi to the implementation of the stitching algorithm.

As this project is a proof of concept, the system presents some limitations, such as the wardrobe small size. This hindrance allows only the use of small garments and a reduced number of clothing items inside at the same time. After testing the system with the small wardrobe, the goal is to validate the complete system with a higher wardrobe capable of allocating larger garments.

Based on the automatic wardrobe developed and the integration with the mobile application *MyEyes*, the final mechatronic system will propose a concept of wardrobe which allows an improvement of blind people's daily routine, specifically in garments identification and management.

Acknowledgment. This work has the support of Association of the Blind and Amblyopes of Portugal (ACAPO) and Association of Support for the Visually Impaired of Braga (AADVDB). Their considerations allow the first insights to a viable solution for the blind people community. This work has been supported by FCT – Fundação para a Ciência e Tecnologia within the R&D Units Project Scope: UIDB/00319/2020.

References

1. Rocha, D., Carvalho, V., Oliveira, E.: MyEyes – automatic combination system of clothing parts to blind people: prototype validation. SENSORDEVICES' 2017 Conference. Rome, Italy 10 – 14 September 2017 (2017)
2. Rocha, D., Carvalho, V., Soares, F., Oliveira, E.: A model approach for an automatic clothing combination system for blind people. In: Brooks, E.I., Brooks, A., Sylla, C., Møller, A.K. (eds.) DLI 2020. LNICSSITE, vol. 366, pp. 74–85. Springer, Cham (2021). https://doi.org/10.1007/978-3-030-78448-5_6
3. Rocha, D., Carvalho, V., Gonçalves, J., et al.: Development of an automatic combination system of clothing parts for blind people: MyEyes. Sens. Transducers **219**, 26–33 (2018)
4. Perry, A.: Consumers' acceptance of smart virtual closets. J. Retail. Consum. Serv. **33**, 171–177 (2016)
5. Rocha, D., Carvalho, V., Soares, F., Oliveira, E., Leão, C.P.: Understand the importance of garments' identification and combination to blind people. In: Ahram, T., Taiar, R. (eds.) IHIET 2021. LNNS, vol. 319, pp. 74–81. Springer, Cham (2022). https://doi.org/10.1007/978-3-030-85540-6_10
6. Rocha, D., Carvalho, V., Soares, F., Oliveira, E.: Design of a mechatronic system to combine garments for blind people: first insights. In: Conference: HealthyIoT 2019 – 6th EAI International Conference on IoT Technologies for HealthCareAt: Braga (2019a)
7. Alabduljabbar, R.: An IoT smart clothing system for the visually impaired using NFC technology. Int. J. Sensor Networks **38**(1), 46–57 (2022)
8. Gatis Filho, S.J.V., de Assumpção Macedo, J., Saraiva, M.M., Souza, J.E.A., Breyer, F.B., Kelner, J.: My best shirt with the right pants: improving the outfits of visually impaired people with QR codes and NFC tags. In: Marcus, A., Wang, W. (eds.) DUXU 2018. LNCS, vol. 10919, pp. 543–556. Springer, Cham (2018). https://doi.org/10.1007/978-3-319-91803-7_41
9. Goh, K.N., Chen, Y.Y., Lin, E.S.: Developing a smart wardrobe system. In: 2011 IEEE Consumer Communications and Networking Conference (CCNC), pp. 303–307 (2011)
10. Official Website. https://www.amazon.com/gp/help/customer/display.html?nodeId=202120810. Accessed October 2022
11. Official Website: https://fashiontasteapi.com/our-technology/. Accessed October 2022
12. Official Website. https://smartcloset.me/. Accessed October 2022
13. Official Website. http://www.tailortags.com/. Accessed October 2022
14. https://www.ikea.com/pt/pt/p/baggebo-armario-c-porta-branco-60481204/. Accessed October 2022

Heart Rate Evaluation by Smartphone:
An Overview

Mohamad Issam Sayyaf$^{(\boxtimes)}$ ⓘ, Domenico Luca Carnì ⓘ, and Francesco Lamonaca ⓘ

University of Calabria, 87036 Arcavacata Di Rende, Italy
f.lamonaca@dimes.unical.it

Abstract. In this paper, an overview of the smartphone measurement methods for Heart Rate (HR) and Heart Rate Variability (HRV) is presented. HR and HRV are important vital signs to be evaluated and monitored especially in a sudden heart crisis and in the case of COVID-19. Unlike other specific medical devices, the smartphone can always be present with a person, and it is equipped with sensors that can be used to estimate or acquire such vital signs. Furthermore, their computation and connection capabilities make them suitable for Internet of Things applications. Although in the literature many interesting solutions for evaluating HR and HRV are proposed, often a lack in the analysis of the measurement uncertainty, the description of the measurement procedure for their validation, and the use of a common gold standard for testing all of them is highlighted. The lack of standardization in experimental protocol, processing methodology, and validation procedures, impacts the comparability of results and their general validity. To stimulate the research activities to fill this gap, the paper gives an analysis of the most recent literature together with a logical classification of the measurement methods by highlighting their main advantages and disadvantages from a metrological point of view together with the description of the measurement methods and instruments proposed by authors for their validation.

Keywords: Heart Rate · Heart Rate Variability · Measurements · Smartphone · Evaluation · Internet of Things (IoT) · Internet of Medical Things (IoMT)

1 Introduction

Heart rate (HR) and heart rate variability (HRV) are important factors for indicating overall health and fitness. In fact, it depends on several physiological and psychological conditions and varies with the variation of this condition. Moreover, they are one of the main parameters to be monitored in the case of COVID-19 [1]. These parameters are usually measured by medically trained staff, but in some specific situations such as for people suffering from tachycardia or bradycardia, continuous monitoring is important. In fact, by defining "tachycardia" as the consistently high resting HR over 100 bpm, this disease is correlated with increased risk for cardiovascular diseases, and it can even be a sign of an underlying heart condition as explained by Dr. Bindu Chebrolu, a cardiologist at Houston Methodist [2]. Increased HR at rest may result in increased

© ICST Institute for Computer Sciences, Social Informatics and Telecommunications Engineering 2023
Published by Springer Nature Switzerland AG 2023. All Rights Reserved
S. Spinsante et al. (Eds.): HealthyIoT 2022, LNICST 456, pp. 14–25, 2023.
https://doi.org/10.1007/978-3-031-28663-6_2

work by the heart, as well as indicating an issue with other physiological pathways. If the HR is closer to 150 bpm or higher, this may be indicative of a condition such as Supraventricular Tachycardia (SVT) requiring medical attention.

A resting heart rate below 60 bpm is considered "bradycardia", but maybe common, particularly in individuals with good cardiovascular fitness or individuals taking certain medications. But sometimes bradycardia can be caused by damage to heart tissues from heart disease or heart attack or inflammatory diseases, such as rheumatic fever or lupus, and can be dangerous [3].

Several portable commercial devices are available in the market for continuous monitoring of HR, such as an oximeter, smartwatch, and smart bracelet. These devices are nowadays smart objects often included on the Internet of Medical Things (IoMT)-based biomedical measurement systems for healthcare monitoring [4]. However, they are adjunctive hardware to manage and carry on. Instead, a device that anyone has always had on himself/herself is the smartphone, and in [5] the authors have proposed an overview of possible applications of smartphones to measure health parameters including blood oxygenation [6] or blood pressure [7].

With the aim to stimulate scientific research, in this paper, we present an overview of the most recent work presented in the literature proposing methods to use the smartphone for measuring HR. Indeed, 83.40% of the world's population owns a smartphone [8].

The main HR measurement can be classified into two categories as shown in (Fig. 1), which are contact and contactless measurements.

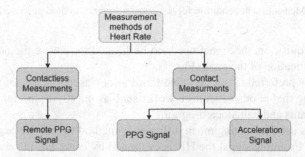

Fig. 1. A classification of measurement methods for heart rate evaluation by smartphone.

Contact measurements are mainly based on the acquisition of the photoplethysmography signal (PPG) or acceleration signal. Contactless measurements are based on the acquisition of a remote PPG signal. In particular, the PPG signal is analysed by time or frequency domain methods, and an automatic classifier. Each method offers advantages and disadvantages, especially concerning measurement accuracy. The critical overview of this method is presented by highlighting the main causes of accuracy degradation and the magnitude of factors influencing the HR measurement.

The paper is organized as follows. In Sect. 2 the measurement method based on contact measurements is presented. In Sect. 3 the measurement method based on contactless measurements is analysed. Finally, some conclusions.

2 Contact-Based Measurement Methods

In contact methods acceleration signals and PPG signals are used to evaluate the HR.

Concerning the first kind of signal, Khairuddin et al. propose a methodology to measure HR and HRV by smartphone depending on the acceleration sensor embedded in a smartphone [9]. The smartphone is placed on the user's chest near the heart and acquires the z-axis signal of the accelerometer. The user must wear light clothing and ·must be in a supine body position as shown in (Fig. 2).

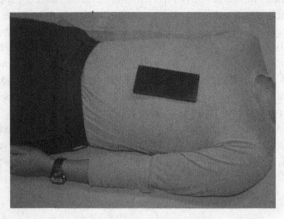

Fig. 2. Measurement condition for the accelerometric method proposed in [9]

After the acquisition, the signal needs to be filtered to remove the noise and make. easier the identification of the peak (Fig. 3).

Although we preferred to use the same terminology as that in the seminal work [9], it is worth noting that in other literature works such as in [10] thesis signals are named seismocardiograms and ballistocardiograms.

The Authors use the moving mean differences method to find the peak value in the signal [11, 12]. From the signal the HR is evaluated by using Eq. (1) and the HRV by monitoring the heartbeat interval RR evaluated by Eq. (2).

$$HR = \frac{number\ of\ heartbeat \times 60}{time\ taken[s]} \tag{1}$$

$$RR_n = t_{HB_n} - t_{HB_{n-1}} \tag{2}$$

where the t_{HB_n} is the time of the nth times of the peak of the heartbeat (R-wave).

The HRV is calculated by computing the standard deviation of RR by using Eq. (3).

$$HRV = \sqrt{\frac{1}{N} \sum_{n=0}^{N-1} (RR_n - \overline{RR_n})^2} \tag{3}$$

The method is experimentally tested by the Authors in 3 experiments on 3 young healthy male students. The age of the students is in the range of 22–25 years old.

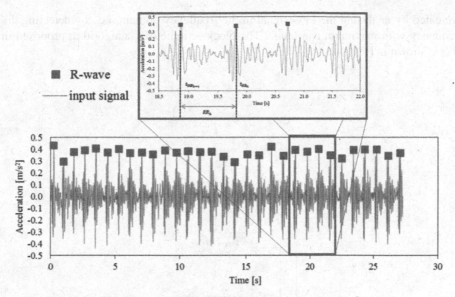

Fig. 3. Acceleration signal with peak value (R-wave)

They compared the results from their proposed method with the result taken by electrocardiogram (ECG).

The experimental results show a maximum difference between the smartphone results and the one achieved with the ECG device equal to 1 bpm. The maximum difference between the HRV evaluated with their proposal and the ECG device is 4 ms.

Dspite these results, the number of experiments is not sufficient to provide a valid statistic. Moreover, the young age of the participants does not allow to test the proposal in the case of heart diseases, tachycardia, bradycardia, or stiffness of the cardiovascular system (typical for elderly people).

As a concern, the measurement method itself, tight or thick clothes can attenuate the accelerometric signal decreasing the (Signal to Noise Ratio) SNR and the measurement accuracy. The method can be ameliorated by a pre-analysis of the acquired signal for evaluating the SNR and checking whether it is suitable for successive steps. Further causes that can misstate the measurement and increase the uncertainty are related to signal artifacts due to movements. Techniques based on automatic classification can be applied to recognize this case and give an alarm about the reliability of the measurements.

Sukaphat et al. [13] propose a methodology to measure HR from the PPG acquired by using the smartphone camera to catch the light emitted by the (Light-emitting diode) LED flash and reflected by the blood in the fingertip. The method was previously proposed by Lamonaca and all in [14].

The fingertip is preliminarily positioned on the smartphone camera to capture the frame's image. Successively, the colour in the captured frame is converted from YUV to RGB format and the PPG value is achieved as the mean value of the red channel. It should be noted that the proposed method considered the correct placement of the finger by using the measurement method proposed by Lamonaca et al. [15]. The HR is evaluated by analysing the PPG signal in the frequency domain, i.e., by detecting the frequency with maximum amplitude. The block scheme of the algorithm proposed in [12] is shown in (Fig. 4).

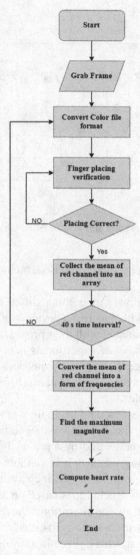

Fig. 4. Flowchart of the algorithm proposed in [12].

The proposed method was tested by 10 people both male and female aged between 20 to 22 years old and with weights between (42 to 88) kg. The results of the proposed method and the results taken from the digital blood pressure were different on average by 0.57%. Furthermore, the p-value for students t-test value is 0.237 that which is greater than the chosen alpha value equal to 0.05. So, the null hypothesis that the heart rate measured by the method proposed by the Authors has the same meaning as the ones achieved by using the gold standard with a trust of 95% can be accepted.

Despite this result, it must be highlighted that the number and the typology of people used in the experiments are not sufficient to evaluate a valid statistic. They did not include old people and people with heart problems or bradycardia and tachycardia, as clearly shown in the experimental results (always in the range (60; 100) bpm, except for one case with the subject with an HR equal to 56 bpm that can be normal for a sportive healthy young subject). Moreover, they should declare how they acquire the data since the cuff for the blood pressure monitor can alter the PPG signal [14]. Finally, the synchronization of the PPG acquisition with the blood pressure monitor is not considered.

Also, Devaki et al. [16] suggested a system to measure the heart rate by using PPG using the mobile phone as a data acquisition device by using the camera and LED flash.

The methodology preliminarily records the video for the fingertip by the camera for 30 s then sends the data to MATLAB to process it. The main steps of the recorded video are:

(i) finding the mean values of the red channel of each frame,
(ii) collect all the values achieving the PPG signal,
(iii) filtering the obtained signal by using bandpass 8th order Butterworth filter in the frequencies (0.8, 7.0) Hz,
(iv) evaluating the Power Spectral Density (PSD),
(v) find the frequency with the maximum amplitude as HR.

The Authors compared their results with the results measured by using a pulse oximeter. The p-value for students t-test value is 0.6 which shows that the readings from the pulse oximeter and smartphone are similar to those values measured for normal and hypertensive patients. Despite this result, the Authors did not give enough information about their experiments, for example, age, sex, and a more comprehensive analysis of the error they achieve, when and why they achieve the maximum error should be interesting. For example, in the case of a normal subject, an error of 8 bpm occurs for an HR equal to 60, which should represent a good case. An error equal to 23 bpm is shown for HR equal to 105, in the case of the Hypertensive subject. Finally, also in this case 10 healthy patients and 10 hypertensive patients seem to be a small sample.

Sabatini et al. also propose a methodology to measure HR and HRV by smartphone depending on the PPG [17]. With respect to the previous method, they use a second-order Butterworth high-pass filter with a cut-off frequency of 0.5 Hz. A further difference is a method for detecting the peak value of the PPG in the time domain based on the Pan-Tompkins algorithm. The HR is the average value of the peak-to-peak distances recorded in 30 s divided by 60.

To evaluate this method the Authors compared it with the results achieved by the Apple watch and used r^2 statistics to achieve information about the goodness of the linear interpolation of the points having as x value the apple watch measurement and y value their method measurement results. It is interesting to note that the Authors present a study showing the influence of the colour channel on the PPG signal, and also in this case red and green channel seems more suitable with respect to the blue one concerning the SNR. Moreover, the Authors highlighted the problem introduced by movement and bad positioning of the finger on the camera. However, in this case, only 8 subjects were used with no information about their health conditions.

Ayesha et al. suggested a system to measure the HR by using PPG acquired by a smartphone camera and elaborate on this signal by using a Convolutional Neural Network (CNN) [18]. In this case, after acquiring the video of the fingertip with the smartphone camera, the average value of each frame channel is detected, and three signals are achieved. Then, the signals are filtered to increase their SNR and a detrending filter is applied to remove the stationary components. Then the signals are normalized by dividing them by their maximum absolute values. The next step is the enhancement by applying a (3x3) kernel moving average filter. Principal Component Analysis was applied to map the source signal into eigenvectors. The first eigenvector is the component with the highest variance, and therefore it was chosen as the PPG signal and a bandpass filter was used to attenuate frequencies outside the range of (0.4, 4.0) Hz that corresponds to (20, 240) bpm. This latter signal is used as input to the CNN. The network consists of 4 convolution layers with ReLU as an activation function and batch normalization and a final fully connected regression layer. The output is the HR given in bpm as shown in (Fig. 5).

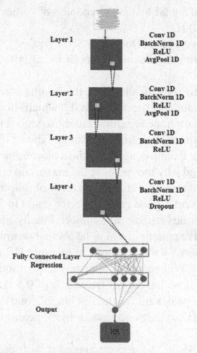

Fig. 5. Neural Network Architecture proposed in [18].

The network was pre-trained using a publicly available PPG-BP dataset [19], containing 657 PPG signal samples collected from 219 subjects by using a finger PPG sensor, together with HR, systolic BP and diastolic BP recorded simultaneously. Using the signal skewness metric, the poor signal samples were discarded [20]. Each sample contains 2100 data points. The sample was clipped to 1800 datapoints and segmented into 3 subparts. Each subpart became an input to the network.

The network was trained for 15 epochs with an SGD optimizer and a learning rate of 0.00001.

They were fine-tuned on a dataset consisting of 51 samples where videos of fingertips were recorded with the Redmi Note 8 smartphone camera. Data were collected from 24 participants, both male and female in the age group of 5 to 77 years. The Authors did not declare, in this case, how they measure the reference values.

The evaluation of the model by using the test data (i.e., the dataset available in [19]) gives a Mean Absolute Error (MAE) of 7.01 bpm and an error percentage of 8.3%. This value is comparable with the error achieved by other methods that do not use artificial intelligence and so can be implemented in the smartphone probably more easily.

The dataset used in this paper is more significant with respect to the ones used in the previously discussed paper both as concerning cardinality and heterogeneity. Unfortunately, a deep discussion about the reason for some significant difference between the estimated HR and the true value (more than 10 bpm in 4 cases, and the maximum difference is 21 bpm) is not given. Further data that should be reported is the clinical history of the people used to build the dataset.

3 Contactless Measurement Methods

Qiao et al. suggested a system to measure the (HR) and (HRV) by using PPG signal extracted from the video of the person's face. This technique is contactless, and it uses the smartphone camera [21, 22].

The main idea is that part of the light is absorbed by the skin, and the rest is reflected. The intensity of the reflected signal is proportional to the blood volume flowing through the tissues. The evaluation of the blood volume over in time is the PPG. The workflow for this method is shown in (Fig. 6) it consists of five stages. The first stage is to detect the Region of Interest (ROI). It is in the face near the nose because it is full of blood vessels, and it is not affected by nose shape and eye movement. The next stage is to acquire the PPG signal correlated with each color for each frame and calculated the average, from (Fig. 6) the green color has the highest value, so the proposed method deals just with the green color. The third stage is signal processing, to remove noise due to movement and handshaking artifacts. In the fourth stage, the peak detection algorithm is applied to calculate the HRV as the temporal difference between two peak occurrences.

In the last stage, the Power Spectral Density (PSD) is applied to the signal to estimate the HR.

To calculate the HR, a band pass filter with cutting frequency of (2.0, 5.0) Hz is applied to the PPG then the PSD is evaluated by using Welch's method [23], and the HR is computed by using the Eq. (4). It is evaluated in pulse per minute (ppm)

$$HR = 60 \times f_{HR} \qquad (4)$$

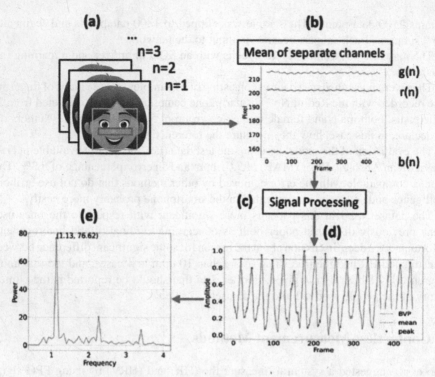

Fig. 6. Overall workflow. (a) Detect face and extract RoI. (b) Calculate the mean of separate channels in every frame and extract the raw BVP signal (g(n)). (c) Process the raw BVP signal with multiple filters to get the final BVP. (d) Detect the peaks of the BVP signal for HRV calculation. (e) Calculate the PSD of BVP in frequency domain for HR calculation [21]. In the pictures, the amplitude values come from pixel intensity. The frequency is in Hz.

The HRV is calculated by finding the interval heartbeats $IBI_n = t_n - t_{n-1}$ where t_n is the time of the nth detected peak. So HRV is calculated by finding the Root Mean Square of Successive IBI Differences [24] as shown in Eq. (5).

$$HRV = \sqrt{\frac{1}{N-1} \sum_{i=1}^{N-1} (IBI_i - IBI_{i+1})^2} \qquad (5)$$

where N is the number of frames.

To evaluate the method, the Authors used a publicly available dataset named "TokyoTech Remote PPG Dataset" [25] consisting of 9 people (8 male and 1 female) for each one of them 3 videos were acquired for testing three situations: relax, exercise, and relax. The video length is 1 min. The proposed method is characterized by MAE equal to 1.49 ± 2.20 bpm for HR and 24.33 ± 28.66 ms for HRV.

Although the cardinality of the testbed seems not too big, and a lack of information about the health status of people is evident, the method shows potentiality for a reliable HR evaluation, and this is important especially in pandemic times. Indeed, the contactless method reduces the risk of contact between the operator and the subject and reduces the time and costs to sanitize the smartphone at each measurement. Experimental results suggest also that possible research should be devoted to ameliorating the HRV evaluation since the variability of the error is comparable with the error itself, which is more than 20% of the measurement.

4 Conclusions

Smartphone are a pervasive tool, i.e., typically anyone has at least one of them always with him/her, also during the night. Thanks to embedded sensors, to their computational capability, and connectivity, the smartphone can be considered a powerful device able to acquire biological signals, evaluate vital signs, and transmit them in the cloud for the online monitoring of patients by clinicians or for self-monitoring.

Heart Rate (HR) and Hearth Rate Variability (HRV) are important vital signs to be monitored in sudden heart crises, stress, and in the case of COVID-19.

Since, unlike other specific medical devices, the smartphone can always be present with a person, this paper the potentiality of the smartphone as a measurement instrument to evaluate HR and HRV without using other adjunctive hardware is investigated.

The overview has highlighted both contact and contactless method to evaluate the HR and HRV. The acquired signals are the PPG acquired by using the camera and the acceleration signal acquired using the accelerometer. The processing methods is based on elaboration in the time domain and frequency domain or by using a Neural Network.

Despite all these research efforts holding a high potential, from this investigation, it was highlighted that a lack of standardization in the experimental protocol, such as how to choose the best location of the smartphone on the body, how to filter and analyze the signal, and how to report the comparison of the results with an accepted gold standard technique, could limit clinical acceptability and prevent recommending this approach as a self-tracking tool, as patient-obtained data quality could be prejudiced. A further main weakness of the research is represented by the fact that reported results are often derived from the observations of few subjects with normal HR and HRV, thus limiting their validity. Also, a lack of knowledge of the technical characteristics of the embedded sensors or of the smartphone itself could impact the evaluation of the HR and HRV measurement uncertainty.

These limitations could be a starting point for future research lines focused to define common test methodologies, gold standards, nomenclature, in order to give a common metrological basis for the comparison of the results achieved with the many methods nowadays available and transforming the common smartphone into a device able to acquire in a simple and non-invasive way, without using any additional hardware, physiological signals and reliable and validated clinical parameters.

Acknowledgement. This research is co-financed by Progetto "Laboratorio Regionale di Ateneo per la Nanomedicina di Precisione Applicata all'Oncologia e alle Malattie Infettive (COVID -19) NLHT-Nanoscience Laboratory for Human Technologies" (ex DGR 459/2020, Asse: - Azione 10.5.12, POR Calabria FESR-FSE 14/20) CUP: J29J14001440007" (DR n. 1410 del 13/10/2021).

References

1. HealthDirect. How to Monitor COVID-19 Symptoms, https://www.healthdirect.gov.au/covid-19/how-to-monitor-symptoms
2. HOUSTON Methodist 6 Sep 2022. https://www.houstonmethodist.org/blog/articles/2021/apr/what-should-your-resting-heart-rate-be/#:~:text=A%20healthy%20heart%20is%20a,efficiently%20as%20it%20could%20be
3. Mayo Clinic 6 Sep 2022. https://www.mayoclinic.org/diseases-conditions/bradycardia/symptoms-causes/syc-20355474#:~:text=Bradycardia%20can%20be%20caused%20by,at%20birth%20(congenital%20heart%20defect)
4. Ahmed, I., Balestrieri, E., Lamonaca, F.: IoMT-Based Biomedical Measurement Systems for Healthcare Monitoring: A Review. **10**(2), 174–184 (2021). Acta IMEKO
5. Polimeni, G., et al.: Health parameters monitoring by smartphone for quality of life improvement. Measurement **73**, 82–94 (2015)
6. Lamonaca, F., et al.: Blood oxygen saturation measurement by smartphone camera. IEEE Intern.Symp.on Medical Measurements and Applications, Italy, pp.359–363 (2015)
7. Van Moer, W., et al.: Photoplethysmogram-based blood pressure evaluation using kalman filtering and neural networks. IEEE Intern.Symp.on Medical Measurements and Applications (MeMeA 2013), Canada, pp. 170–174 (2013)
8. Bank my cell 6 Sep 2022. https://www.bankmycell.com/blog/how-many-phones-are-in-the-world
9. Khairuddin M.K.N.B., Nakamoto, K., Nakamura, H., Tanaka, K., Nakashima, S.: Heart rate and heart rate variability measuring system by using smartphone. In: 5th International Conference on Applied Computing and Information Technology/4th Intl Conference on Computational Science/Intelligence and Applied Informatics/2nd International Conference on Big Data, Cloud Computing, Data Science (ACIT-CSII-BCD), pp. 47–52 (2017)
10. Landreani, F., Caiani, E.G.: Smartphone Accelerometers for the Detection of Heart Rate. Expert Review of Medical Devices. **14**(12), 935–948 (2017). https://doi.org/10.1080/17434440.2017.1407647
11. Scholkmann, F., Boss, J., Martin, W.: An efficient algorithm for automatic peak detection in noisy periodic and quasi-periodic signals. Algorithms **5**(4), 588–603 (2012)
12. Yang, C., He, Z., Yu, W.: Comparison of public peak detection algorithms for MALDI mass spectrometry data analysis. BMC Bioinformatics **10**(1), 1–13 (2009)
13. Sukaphat, S., Nanthachaiporn, S., Upphaccha, K., Tantipatrakul, P.: Heart rate measurement on android platform. In: 13th International Conference on Electrical Engineering/Electronics, Computer, Telecommunications and Information Technology (ECTI-CON), pp. 1–5 (2016)
14. Lamonaca, F., Kurylyak, Y., Grimaldi, D., Spagnuolo, V.: Reliable pulse rate evaluation by smartphone. In: IEEE International Symposium on Medical Measurements and Applications Proceedings, pp. 1–4 (2012)
15. Grimaldi, D., Kurylyak, Y., Lamonaca, F., Nastro, A.: Photoplethysmography detection by smartphone's videocamera. In: Proceedings of the 6th IEEE International Conference on Intelligent Data Acquisition and Advanced Computing Syst. **1**, pp. 488–491 (2011)
16. Devaki, V., Jayanthi, T.: Pulse rate measurement using android smartphone. In: International Conference on Wireless Communications Signal Processing and Networking (WiSPNET), pp. 22–25 (2019)
17. Sabatini, A., Iannello, G., Pennazza, G., Santonico, M., Spinosa, M., Vollero, L.: Heart rate analysis through smartphone camera. In: IEEE International Workshop on Metrology for Industry 4.0 & IoT (MetroInd4.0&IoT), pp. 402–406 (2021)
18. Ayesha, A.H., Qiao, D., Zulkernine, F.: Heart rate monitoring using PPG with smartphone camera. In: IEEE International Conference on Bioinformatics and Biomedicine (BIBM), pp. 2985–2991 (2021)

19. Liang, Y., Liu, G., Chen, Z., Elgendi, M.: PPG-BP Database (2018). https://doi.org/10.6084/m9.figshare.5459299. Accessed 25 Sep 2021
20. Chowdhury, M., et al.: Estimating blood pressure from the photoplethysmogram signal and demographic features Using machine learning techniques. Artificial Intelligence in Medical Sensors, MDPI (2020)
21. Qiao, D., Zulkernine, F., Masroor, R., Rasool, R., Jaffar, N.: Measuring heart rate and heart rate variability with smartphone camera. In: 2021 22nd IEEE International Conference on Mobile Data Management (MDM), pp. 248–249 (2021)
22. Spagnolo, G.S., Cozzella, L., Leccese, F.: Project of electronic identity of painting. Paper presented at the 2020 IMEKO TC-4 International Conference on Metrology for Archaeology and Cultural Heritage, pp. 420–424 (2020)
23. Welch, P.: The use of fast Fourier transforms for the estimation of power spectra: a method based on time averaging over short, modified periodograms. IEEE Transactions on audio and Electroacoustics 15(2), 70–73 (1967)
24. Shaffer, F., Ginsberg, J.P.: An overview of heart rate variability metrics and norms. Front. Public Health 5, 258 (2017)
25. Maki, S., Monno, Y., Yoshizaki, K., Tanaka, M., Okutomi, M.: Inter beat inter-val estimation from facial video based on reliability of BVP signals. In: 41st Annual International Conference of the IEEE Engineering in Medicine and Biology Society (EMBC), pp. 6525–6528 (2019)

A Low-Cost Open-Source Bionic Hand Controller: Preliminary Results and Perspectives

Sandra Rodrigues[1] and Milton P. Macedo[1,2](✉) 📷

[1] Instituto Politécnico de Coimbra, ISEC, DFM, Rua Pedro Nunes, Quinta da Nora, 3030-199 Coimbra, Portugal
mpmacedo@isec.pt
[2] Department of Physics, LIBPhys, University of Coimbra, Rua Larga, 3004-516 Coimbra, Portugal

Abstract. This paper presents the current state of an ongoing project for the implementation of a low-cost bionic hand controller. Research had been conducted to evaluate the possibility of using MechanoMyoGraphic signals (MMG) as an alternative to ElectroMyoGraphic signals (EMG) that are usually acquired. Moreover the application of two novel and low-cost electrodes, one built from a conductive leather material, and another based on desktop 3D printing using conductive PLA (PolyLactic Acid), as an alternative to traditional pre-gelled Ag/AgCl electrodes was also evaluated. In addition to the search for the optimization of the quality of acquired signals, a solution for the control of the bionic hand had also been implemented using a very low-cost microcontroller (Arduino UNO). Results will be briefly presented from these works already carried out. A particular emphasis should be given to the success rate attained of 100% on detecting three out of four gestures selected, when using this very low-cost hardware platform. However false activations were a weakness of this solution. In order to optimize bionic hand control, the simultaneous application of three types of sensors (EMG, force and accelerometer) is ongoing. A description of this implementation as well as a presentation of its preliminary results will also be made.

Keywords: Electromyography (EMG) · Mechanomyography (MMG) · Bionic hand · Biomedical sensors · Feature extraction

1 Introduction

The field of hand prostheses is under continuous evolution because of huge research constantly being developed in order to improve the quality in the way they reproduce the functionalities of the human hand, but also in the search for more economical solutions. It is a typical area of biomedical engineering since, in addition to the knowledge of the anatomy of the forearm and hand muscles as well as of the electromyographic signals involved, it also encompasses the knowledge of physics, mathematics and engineering

S. Spinsante et al. (Eds.): HealthyIoT 2022, LNICST 456, pp. 26–39, 2023.
https://doi.org/10.1007/978-3-031-28663-6_3

areas, which are demanded for the acquisition of signals and their processing. The advancement of 3D printing technologies this will also be an important area for the production of the low-cost prostheses itself.

Unlike myoelectric prostheses in which the opening and closing of the hand is made without individualized control of each finger, the bionic hands have a controller that, by collecting the myoelectric signal in one or more muscles, discriminates gestures through feature extraction and with the help of machine learning techniques.

This work aims to address only one of the strands that contributes to the success of bionic hands and that is the improvement of the quality of the acquired signal, with a view to the implementation of a low-cost bionic hand.

In spite of the typical approach of using EMG signals, there are some drawbacks that have led to the attempts of extracting other type of information, namely to predict muscle forces from EMG signals using the wavelet transform [1]. One of these drawbacks is the fact that EMG signals are often degraded due to electromagnetic interference and implies a large amount of processing time for features extraction [2].

In contrast, the mechanical change of the muscles can be measured by a method with sensitivity to the position / motion of a small area in surface of the muscle, and is typically known as MMG (MechanoMyography). Different type of sensors had been used in several studies reported in literature, since the application of microphones and/or accelerometers [3–6] through force sensors [2] or even light detectors, namely IR (InfraRed) sensors [7, 8], in an individual manner or some of them together even with also EMG sensors [9–12].

In this work, preliminary results of the application of MMG sensors, such as FSR (Force Sensitive Resistor) and IR sensors with the BITalino (Plux Biosignals) platform have already been obtained [13]. It has also been studied the possibility of applying of its EMG sensor module with two novel and low-cost electrodes: one built from a conductive leather material, and another based on desktop 3D printing using conductive PLA (PolyLactic Acid), by comparison with pre-gelled Ag/AgCl electrodes, considered as the reference electrode [14].

This paper will summarize these studies and their preliminary results. Firstly it is presented the evaluation of the application of MMG sensors as an alternative to traditional EMG and then the evaluation of the application of new electrodes more economical and reusable as an alternative to traditional pre-gelled Ag/AgCl. It will also feature the low-cost platform based on Arduino Uno which was developed for bionic hand control, using only EMG signals. For this implementation, an onset/offset design algorithm was developed to meet the requirements of real-time control and the limitations of memory space and processing speed of this low-cost microcontroller [15]. Finally, the platform that is currently being implemented will be described. It is based on the integration of MMG (FSR and accelerometer) and EMG sensors with the aim of optimizing the quality of the acquired signal and thus the success rate of the bionic hand controller.

2   Study of Mechanomyographic Alternatives to EMG Sensors

A comparative study was made of the application of a FSR and a IR sensor with the reference signal in the scope of this work, the EMG signal [13]. A summary of the main specifications of these three sensors can be found in Table 1.

Table 1. Main specifications of each sensor.

EMG Module specifications	
Gain	1000
Range	± 1.65 mV
Bandwidth	10-400 Hz
FSR 400 Specifications	
Force Sensitivity Range	0.110.0 N
Force Repeatability	± 2%
Number of actuations (life time)	10 million
QTR-1A Reflectance Sensor Specifications	
Optimal Sensing Distance	3 mm
Maximum Sensing Distance	6 mm

The acquisition of the signals from each sensor is performed through the hardware platform BITalino Plugged; its OpenSignals software enables real-time data acquisition and recording in a CSV (Comma-Separated Values) format. These data is subsequently used in MATLAB (MathWorks ®) for data processing and analysis.

Besides the BITalino EMG sensor it was then used a force sensor in order to react to changes in the muscle volumes, for which an FSR 400 sensor (Interlink Electronics, USA) was selected. A third sensor was used in this study to extract features related with the variations in light reflected at the skin surface, as a result of the changes in muscle volume due to the contraction. For the acquisition of this data, a QTR-1A reflectance sensor (Pololu Corporation, USA) was used. It includes an IR LED (Light Emitting Diode) and a phototransistor, and the output varies proportionally to the amount of light reflected on a surface.

An extremely important issue for the acquisition of signals from any of these three sensors, with a fair signal-to-noise ratio and appropriate sensitivity, is a correct placement of the sensors. Photos of the placement of each of the three sensors are shown in Fig. 1.

For FSR and IR sensors, raw-data was used in spite of a variable baseline that eventually could be corrected through the use of the derivative of these signals. The EMG sensor is used in a bipolar differential front-end for a higher signal- to-noise ratio. Firstly a bandpass filter was applied to raw-data with a frequency range of 20 to 500 Hz [16]. It is important to cancel the powerline noise, so a bandreject filter is used for the 50–60 Hz range. Figure 2 shows an example of raw-data for each sensor.

For a more objective comparison between those signals, signal-to noise ratio (SNR) which is a quite well established parameter, it was calculated through the ratio of peak-to-peak values of signals from muscle activation periods and of noise from rest period.

Table 2 shows a summary of these SNR results as well as those achieved for onset/offset detection rates and in Table 3 is presented the success rate in gesture identification.

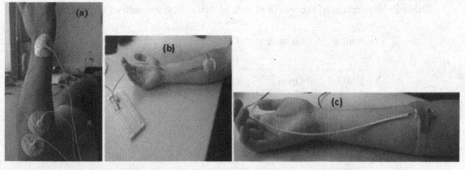

Fig. 1. Photos of the sensors placement. Three EMG pre-gelled electrodes (a), FSR sensor with velcro strap for fixation (b), and IR sensor mounted inside a 3D printed fixation support and velcro strap for fixation (c).

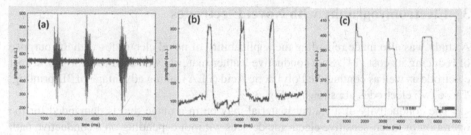

Fig. 2. Example of raw data of each sensor in case of a gesture of close. EMG (a), FSR (b) and IR sensor (c).

Table 2. Summary of SNR analysis and Onset/Offset recognition rates for each of three sensors.

Sensor	Gesture	SNR (dB)	Onset/Offset Detection	
			Detected/Total	(%)
EMG	Open	4.5	54/54	100/
	Close	2.1	70/72	97%
	Point	2.2	23/39	59%
FSR	Open	10.0	39/42	93%
	Close	9.6	87/96	91%
IR	Open	9.1	46/48	96%
	Close	14.0	59/60	98%

For this study each sensor was placed individually and acquisitions were carried out using similar timing parameters. The sampling data was collected from four healthy subjects (2 men, 2 women). In each acquisition, the same gesture was made three times. Each gesture lasts for approximately three seconds with similar rest time between them.

Table 3. Percentage of success in gesture identification for each of three sensors.

Sensor	Gesture	Gesture Identification	
		False/True	(%)
EMG	Open	6/48	89%
	Close	22/48	69%
	Point	2/21	91%
FSR	Open	0/39	100%
	Close	13/74	85%
IR	Open	0/46	100%
	Close	0/59	100%

3 Electromyography with Novel Electrodes

A study was also made regarding the applicability of novel electrodes with the purpose of reducing its cost [14]. So a conductive leather material was used to build a low-cost electrode as well as conductive PolyLactic Acid (PLA) taking advantage of 3D printing. These two electrodes are shown in Fig. 3.

The conductivity of a leather material may be in a range that is demanded for the operation of touch-sensitive electronic devices without depending on a conductive path to the human body. To change its conductivity electrically conductive metallic particles can be incorporated which could allow its application for EMG electrodes.

PLA can be considered cost efficient to produce and it is biodegradable. Amongst a wide set of PLA applications it is already well established its use for biodegradable medical devices. PLA has also the property of melting easily so it is an obvious choice for some interesting applications in 3D printing. In this case it is intended to replace traditional EMG electrodes through its function with conductive properties.

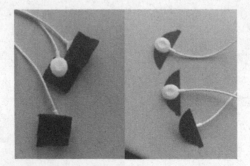

Fig..3. Two novel electrodes. Conductive leather (left) and PLA (right).

The acquisitions from 15 healthy young subjects were carried out using similar timing parameters. The sampling data is summarized in Table 4. Each acquisition contains in average a set of four same gestures executed for around three seconds each and separated by a resting time of similar magnitude. For this study the first choice was to use six different gestures (Open, Close, Point, Pinch, Flexion, Extension).

MATLAB tools were used to perform feature extraction. Amongst others that were initially also considered, a set of six features were selected in order to be evaluated in each muscle activation [17]: Maximum, Minimum, RMS, Mean; Standard deviation, and Peak-to-Peak value. For gesture recognition it was necessary to find an appropriate data science and machine learning platform that should use a dataset that comprises the extracted features i.e. the values of those six features, calculated for each correctly detected muscle activation. These whole data was evaluated in RapidMiner.

Table 4. Description of the whole data acquired: Number of acquisition files (AcqF) and of muscle activations (MAct).

Sensor	Gesture	open		close		flexion[1]		extension[1]		pinch		point	
	Electrodes	AcqF	MAct	AcqF	MAct	AcqF	MAct	AcqF	MAct	AcqF	MAct	AcqF	MAct
EMG	Ag/AgCl	9	37	5	19	6	21	5	18	7	29	9	37
	Leather	12	47	12	59	11	46	8	30	8	32	12	47
	PLA	11	46	8	33	8	34	6	24	8	33	11	46

[1] Entire hand flexion/extension

In order to optimize the success of RapidMiner on gesture recognition it was important to define the ratio of data used for training and data used for evaluating gesture recognition. After some tests the dataset was splitted so that 70% of the whole data was for that training with the purpose of learning how to use the combination of six extracted features to achieve an higher success on the recognition of the six gestures. Consequently the remaining 30% of the data was effectively applied on the prediction of the different gestures. Also the different processing tools provided by RapidMiner were tested from which two (Decision Tree and Neural Network) were used.

As mentioned the initial goal was to perform the gesture recognition for all the six gestures. Unfortunately it was concluded that this amount of data collected from just one sensor and always in the same muscle for all acquisitions was insufficient to succeed. A less ambitious goal was then established that consisted on evaluating the accuracy on the recognition of sets of two, three and four gestures.

Amongst several parameters that RapidMiner computes, accuracy was chosen for this analysis. In fact accuracy is defined as the fraction of whole gestures that are correctly classified (TP + TN). In this manner it describes the overall effectiveness of the classification process. In a more complete way it is given by the ratio of those whole gestures that are correctly classified to the whole data (TP + FP + TN + FN). Figure 4 summarizes graphically those values of accuracy computed in RapidMiner, in order to compare the overall accuracy computed for each sensor/electrode type as well as to compare that accuracy for some gesture combinations.

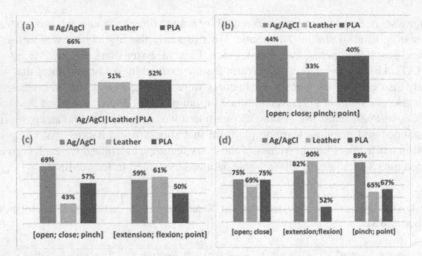

Fig. 4. Bar graphs showing a comparison of the accuracy in gesture recognition between electrode types, for the whole results available (a) and for each gesture combination (b-d).

4 Bionic Hand Controller

The success on the control of a bionic hand depends heavily on success on the identification of gestures. It is then essential to optimize onset/offset detection so that feature extraction is also improved. On the other hand this control requires that, in real time, onset/offset detection is made, as well as feature extraction and consequent identification of gestures. To implement all these features in a microcontroller ATmega328 microprocessor with 16 MHz clock speed and 32 kBytes of memory, an onset/offset detection algorithm was adapted [15]. This controller uses only the EMG signal acquired with pre-gelled Ag/AgCl electrodes. The BITalino EMG sensor was used to acquire these signals. This BITalino platform was used for the simultaneous acquisition and visualization of data in OpenSignals with the purpose of providing a mean for support on the debug of the algorithm running in the Arduino UNO.

The evaluation of the success was carried out using a servo-driven bionic-hand controller prototype, as shown in Fig. 5. Four different gestures were executed: Open, Close, Point and Pinch. Each finger is controlled by a dedicated Micro Servo SG90 (TowerPro). Each gesture is accomplished by an adequate combination of finger activation.

Additional factors were identified that may reduce detection success such as the noise in the EMG signals coming from electromagnetic interference, namely that the different rotation of the servomotors to carry out each finger generates different noise. Noise was also noted as a result of forearm movement artifacts. Due care was taken with regard to noise reduction by reducing the length of cables and winding them up. Even with the conditions presented, the results obtained for different gestures were satisfactory, as shown in Table 5.

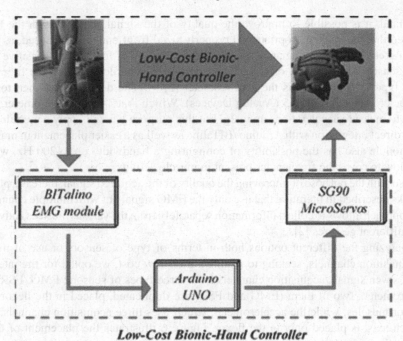

Low-Cost Bionic-Hand Controller

Fig. 5. Scheme of the prototype of the bionic-hand controller.

Table 5. Results of success on detection of muscle activation for the execution of different gestures.

Gesture	close	open	point	pinch
# performed	20	20	20	10
# detected	20	14	20	10
# not detected	0	6	0	0
# false activations	1	4	2	0
Success rate	100%	70%	100%	100%
Error rate	5%	50%	10%	0%

5   Platform with Integration of EMG and MMG Signals

In order to optimize hand control it is essential to improve the quality of the information acquired, as this will enhance the identification of the different gestures. As already mentioned there are numerous studies described in the literature, which have in common the search for sensors that can be used alternatively or in addition to the EMG signal [2–12]. Although the preliminary results presented here show that the IR sensor has a good SNR ratio, similar to or even higher than that of the FSR, it was verified that it has a more limited applicability with regard to the diversity of gestures detected. On the other hand, it is possible to improve the quality of the signal acquired with the FSR, provided that the most appropriate and properly sized front-end circuit is used, as well as with greater care in fixing and ensuring the application of force in the sensitive area of the sensor. Another type of sensor with positive results described in the literature in this type of application is the accelerometer [5, 6]. The decision was then to add the accelerometer ADXL335 (Analog Devices). Which is a 3-axis accelerometer, that allows to measure accelerations up to 3g. For this purpose we will apply a module that allows direct integration with Arduino /BITalino as well as a easier placement in muscle. This module also has the possibility of configuring a bandwidth up to 200 Hz, which will allow to cover the frequencies present in muscle activity.

Also with the purpose of improving the quality of the acquired signal, there is a plenty of works described in literature that use only the EMG signal but with multiple channels. This approach allows to collect information separately from the various muscles activated in the different gestures [2].

Analyzing the different options both in terms of type of sensors or use of multiple acquisition channels, seeking to maintain their low cost, we opted for the integration of seven signals/acquisition channels from three types of sensors: EMG, FSR and accelerometer. Two of them (EMG and FSR) are duplicated, placed in the flexor and extensor muscles, while the accelerometer, which uses three acquisition channels, one for each axis, is placed only in the flexor. Figure 6 illustrates the placement of these sensors/electrodes.

Seven BITalino acquisition channels will then be used, and the data is acquired from a group of volunteers and according to a previously defined protocol. Data processing and feature extraction will be performed on MATLAB. The identification of the different gestures will then be attained from the introduction of the datasets with the characteristics of the seven acquired signals, using one selected data science and machine learning tool.

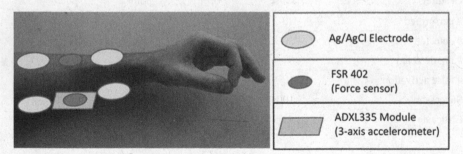

Fig. 6. Scheme of the integration of three type of sensors (EMG, FSR and accelerometer) showing the placement of Ag/AgCl electrodes and FSR in both flexion and extension muscles and accelerometer only in the flexion muscle.

5.1 Preliminary Tests

A first approach to the implementation of these different types of sensors was made using the two force sensors and two EMG sensors, in a total of four acquisition channels. Data were acquired from one ordinary healthy subject that performed five different gestures (*Open*, *Close*, *Pinch*, *Point* and *Thumb-up*). In each acquisition it was always executed the same gesture for ten times with a duration and interval approximately constants.

The data was acquired through four BITalino channels with a 10-bit ADC each. This data was viewed in real-time in Opensignals and later stored in a file for further processing in MATLAB ®. In these preliminary tests, no processing was carried out to the EMG signal and the onset/offset detection of each muscle activation was accomplished from the acquired FSR signal. This was performed separately for the FSR and EMG signals acquired from the flexor muscles and extensor muscles.

This first approach to the integration of these sensors had as main objective to evaluate their advantages over the platform initially used with only one channel of acquisition of an EMG signal. This analysis should be made according to three complementary perspectives:

1. Four signals are acquired through four channels, simultaneously;
2. The signals are of two different types: EMG and MMG;
3. Sensors are placed in two different locations: flexor and extensor muscles.

Using a simple criterion for the validation of onset/offset detection that has had a minimum duration of 0.5 s, the success rate was high, as shown in Table 6.

Table 6. Results of success on detection of muscle activation for the execution of different gestures. Flex and Ext mean Flexor and Extensor muscles, respectively.

Gesture	close		open		point		pinch		thumb-up	
	Flex	Ext	Flex	Ext	Flex	Ext	Flex	Ext	Flex	Ext
# performed	10	10	10	10	10	10	10	10	10	10
# detected	10	10	8	10	10	6	10	7	10	10
# not detected	0	0	2	0	0	4	0	3	0	0
# false activations	0	0	0	0	0	0	0	0	0	0
Success rate	100%	100%	80%	100%	100%	60%	100%	70%	100%	100%
Error rate	0%	0%	20%	0%	0%	40%	0%	30%	0%	0%

Figures 7, 8, 9 show a sample with a period of 20 s relative to the four signals acquired for each of three different gestures chosen amongst the five executed. Figure 7 shows that for the *Open* while the EMG signals acquired in the flexor and extensor muscles are very similar the FSR signal obtained from the extensor muscles has an amplitude that stands out from that relative to flexors.

In opposition to the previous case, Fig. 8 shows that for *Pinch* the amplitude of the acquired FSR signal for the flexor and extensor muscles are very similar. But the complementarity between FSR and EMG signals, associated with different behaviors

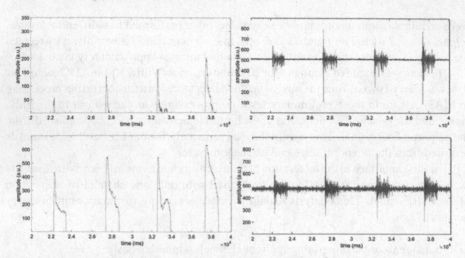

Fig. 7. Four signals acquired from flexor muscles (top) and extensor muscles (bottom) for *Open*. (Left) FSR and (Right) EMG signals.

for different gestures, is a result that meets our expectations and is very useful for the success in gesture recognition.

Finally, and unlike the two previous gestures, in *Thumb-up* the success rate in detecting their activations was 100%. In Fig. 9 it can be observed that the amplitude of the two FSR signals is superior to that of the other two gestures, with a greater amplitude in the case of flexor muscles, in which it is also shown to have a less fluctuating amplitude during activation.

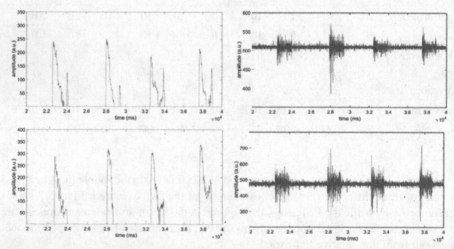

Fig. 8. Four signals acquired from flexor muscles (top) and extensor muscles (bottom) for *Pinch*. (Left) FSR and (Right) EMG signals.

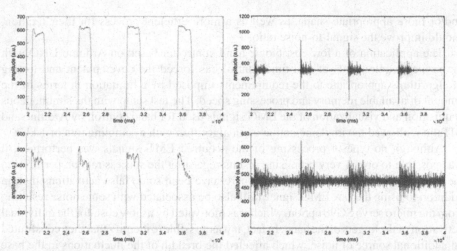

Fig. 9. Four signals acquired from flexor muscles (top) and extensor muscles (bottom) for *Thumb-up*. (Left) FSR and (Right) EMG signals

The mere observation of the signals acquired by these four channels confirms that the amount of information that is available with the consequent characteristics that can be extracted will be an added value for success in gesture recognition. Moreover, with the FSR signals the onset/offset detection becomes easier. In the case of EMG signals, one should look for the characteristics that will contribute the most to this success and which at the same time imply a shorter processing time with a view to its application in a low-cost bionic-hand controller.

6   Discussion and Conclusions

Results of the application of two MMG sensors, a FSR and an IR reflectance sensor, and their comparison with EMG signals have shown successful results in gesture recognition and a high SNR (Signal-to-Noise Ratio). It was also shown a slightly better ability of EMG sensor to detect different gestures, but simultaneously it had a lower success in gesture identification. IR sensors have shown similar results comparatively to FSR in the ability to detect different gestures but an even better success in gesture identification. Also IR and FSR signals had shown higher SNR than traditional EMG signals, for the two gestures that those two sensors were able to detect.

On the other hand the comparison between electrodes types had shown a slightly lower accuracy of the conductive leather and PLA in relation to the common electrodes. Nevertheless the conductive leather material electrodes have shown an improved accuracy in two of the total of six gesture combinations considered.

In spite of their lower overall accuracy in gestures recognition, in comparison to pre-gelled Ag/AgCl electrodes, the results obtained for the novel electrodes are very similar to those traditional EMG electrodes in, at least, half of the six gestures. The exceptions are the point and pinch gestures for conductive leather material, and those plus extension gesture for conductive PLA electrodes. Electrodes with a larger area and/or more appropriate shape, as well as a more efficient process for their fixation, should improve the signal-to-noise ratio.

The application of a low-cost bionic hand controller based on Arduino UNO with the proper requirements of real-time control has forced the development and testing of algorithms appropriate to the requirements imposed by a limitation in terms of the amount of available memory and processing speed. The test setup with the simultaneous acquisition and visualization of the EMG signals used for hand control, by Arduino and BITalino, allowed the implementation of an algorithm with a sampling rate of 1 kHz.

Although no type of processing of the acquired EMG signals was performed, it was possible to obtain very promising results regarding the success rate on performing the four different gestures considered. There have been some false activations that, in addition to using the raw EMG signal, will also be associated with some noise resulting from the micro servo SG90 option, which was motivated by its low cost, for the individual activation of the fingers of the hand. In fact, it was possible to identify that they constituted an additional source of noise, which affected the breadth of the fluctuations in the base level of the signal, with the muscle relaxed, depending on the gesture associated with the previous muscle activation.

Based on these preliminary results and those of other studies described in the literature, we opted for the implementation of a platform that complements EMG signals with two other MMG signals collected by a force sensor and an accelerometer. A next phase of this work is then underway in which these three types of sensors (EMG, FSR and accelerometer) will be integrated, and signals from the flexor and extensor muscles will be collected at the same time, in a total of seven acquisition channels. With this approach it will be possible to minimize the limitations resulting from the interferences to which the EMG signal is subject, maintaining the future possibility of implementing a low-cost controller, even with greater requirements in terms of memory space and processing capacity than the Arduino UNO, used in the preliminary version of the controller. It will be necessary to develop the more demanding algorithm in terms of the acquisition of the different acquisition channels, as well as in their processing, with possible implementation also of EMG signal filtering.

References

1. Wei, G., Tian, F., Tang, G., Wang, C.: A wavelet-based method to predict muscle forces from surface electromyography signals in weightlifting. J. Bionic Eng. **9**, 48–58 (2012)
2. Li, N., Yang, D., Jiang, L., Liu, H., Cai, H.: Combined use of FSR sensor array and SVM classifier for finger motion recognition based on pressure distribution map. J. Bionic Eng. **9**(1), 39–47 (2012)
3. Buk, A.A.Y., et al.: Hand gesture recognition using mechanomyography signal based on LDA classifier. IOP Conf. Series: Materials Science and Eng. **881**(1), 012125 (2020)
4. Wilson, S., Vaidyanathan, R.: Upper-limb prosthetic control using wearable multichannel mechanomyography. IEEE Conference on Rehabilitation Robotics, pp. 1293–1298 (2017)
5. Alves, N., Chau, T.: Uncovering patterns of forearm muscle activity using multi-channel mechanomyography. J. Electromyogr. Kinesiol. **20**(5), 777–786 (2010)
6. Kaczmarek, P., Mańkowski, T., Tomczyński, J.: Towards sensor position-invariant hand gesture recognition using a mechanomyographic interface. Signal Processing: Algorithms, Architectures, Arrangements, and Applications (SPA), pp. 53–58 (2017)

7. Nsugbe, E.: A pilot exploration on the use of NIR monitored haemodynamics in gesture recognition for transradial prosthesis control. Intelligent Systems with Appl. **9**, 200045 (2021)
8. Rohithm, H.R., Gowtham, S., Chandra, A.S.: Hand gesture recognition in real time using IR sensor. International Journal of Pure and Applied Mathematics **114**(7), 111–121 (2017)
9. Wan, B.,. Wu, R., Zhang, K., Liu, L.: A new subtle hand gestures recognition algorithm based on EMG and FSR. IEEE 21st International Conference on Computer Supported Cooperative Work in Design, pp. 127–132 (2017)
10. Esposito, D., et al.: A piezoresistive sensor to measure muscle contraction and mechanomyography. Sensors **18**(8), 2553 (2018)
11. Kawamoto, T., Yamazaki, N.: Bulk movement included in multi-channel mechanomyography: similarity between mechanomyography of resting muscle and that of contracting muscle. J. Electromyogr. Kinesiol. **22**(6), 923–929 (2012)
12. Guo, W., Sheng, X., Liu, H., Zhu, X.: Mechanomyography assisted myoeletric sensing for upper-extremity prostheses: a hybrid approach. IEEE Sens. J. **17**(10), 3100–3108 (2017)
13. Marques, J., Ramos, S., Macedo, M.P., da Silva, H.P.: Study of mechanomyographic alternatives to EMG sensors for a low-cost open source bionic hand. In: Inácio, P.R.M., Duarte, A., Fazendeiro, P., Pombo, N. (eds.) HealthyIoT 2018. EICC, pp. 3–14. Springer, Cham (2020). https://doi.org/10.1007/978-3-030-30335-8_1
14. Silva, D., Castro, S., Macedo, M.P., Silva, H.P.: Towards improving the usability of muscle sensing in open source bionic hand: mechanomyography vs. electromyography with novel electrodes. AmiEs-2019 - International Symposium on Ambient Intelligence and Embedded Systems, pp. 1–6 (2019)
15. Rodrigues, S., Macedo, M.P.: Algorithm for onset/offset detection of EMG signals for real-time control of a low-cost open-source bionic-hand. In: Proceedings of the 15th Int. Joint Conf. on Biomedical Engineering Systems and Technologies – WHC, pp. 872–878 (2022)
16. Balbinot, A., Favieiro, G.: A neuro-fuzzy system for characterization of arm movements. Sensors **13**(2), 2613–2630 (2013)
17. Freitas, M.L.B., et al.: Sistema de extração de caraterísticas do sinal de TM eletromiografia de tempo e frequência em Labview. In: Anais do V Congresso Brasileiro de Eletromiografia e Cinesiologia e X Simpósio de Engenharia Biomédica, Even3 Publisher, pp. 820–823 (2018)

Preliminary Study on Gender Identification by Electrocardiography Data

Eduarda Sofia Bastos[1], Rui Pedro Duarte[1], Francisco Alexandre Marinho[1],
Luís Pimenta[1], António Jorge Gouveia[1], Norberto Jorge Gonçalves[1(✉)],
Paulo Jorge Coelho[2,3], Eftim Zdravevski[4], Petre Lameski[4], Nuno M. Garcia[5],
and Ivan Miguel Pires[5]

[1] Escola de Ciências e Tecnologia, University of Trás-os-Montes e Alto Douro,
Quinta de Prados, 5001-801 Vila Real, Portugal
{al70647,al70650,al171518,al70827}@alunos.utad.pt, {jgouveia,
njg}@utad.pt
[2] Polytechnic of Leiria, 2411-901 Leiria, Portugal
paulo.coelho@ipleiria.pt
[3] Institute for Systems Engineering and Computers at Coimbra (INESC Coimbra),
3030-790 Coimbra, Portugal
[4] Faculty of Computer Science and Engineering, University Ss Cyril and Methodius,
1000 Skopje, Macedonia
{eftim.zdravevski,petre.lameski}@finki.ukim.mk
[5] Instituto de Telecomunicações, Universidade da Beira Interior, 6200-001 Covilhã, Portugal
ngarcia@di.ubi.pt, ivan.pires@lx.it.pt

Abstract. Medical teams can use an electrocardiogram (ECG) as a quick test to examine the electrical activity and rhythm of the heart to look for irregularities that may be indicative of diseases. This work aims to summarize the outcomes of several artificial intelligence techniques developed to identify ECG data by gender automatically. The analysis and processing of ECG data were collected from 219 individuals (112 males, 106 females, and one other) aged between 12 and 92 years in different geographical regions, located mainly in the municipalities of the center of Portugal. These data allowed to discretize gender by the analysis of ECG data during the experiment performed and were acquired with the BITalino (r)evolution device, connected to a personal computer, using the OpenSignals (r)evolution software. The dataset describes the acquisition conditions, the individual's characteristics, and the sensors used as the data acquired from the ECG sensor.

Keywords: ECG · Gender identification · Artificial intelligence · Sensors

1 Introduction

The early detection of cardiovascular issues is essential for reducing the fatality rate associated with cardiovascular diseases [3, 18], which are among the major causes of

S. Spinsante et al. (Eds.): HealthyIoT 2022, LNICST 456, pp. 40–49, 2023.
https://doi.org/10.1007/978-3-031-28663-6_4

death worldwide [6, 27]. For this reason, we believe that experts should adopt automatic electrocardiogram (ECG) analysis to aid in diagnosing cardiovascular diseases [11, 19, 20].

The research on the gender identification is a new subject that is currently starting with more research studies, but the number of studies available in the literature is very small [2, 24]. However, if the studies were performed, we can classify the results according with the gender.

We investigated the most recent machine learning techniques for categorizing and analysis of ECG signals and found that few studies have been unsuccessful in achieving high precision rates [2, 24]. Due to this, we decided to do our research using a dataset we had built and some of the methods we had discovered during our search.

We implemented eight different methods to analyze the results: Nearest Neighbors, Linear SVM, RBF SVM, Decision Tree, Random Forest, Neural Networks, AdaBoost, and Naive Bayes. Based on the machine learning methods, the data was classified by Gender.

2 Methods

2.1 Study Design and Participants

Using a BITalino (r)evolution device [10], and the OpenSignals (r)evolution software, [7], 219 individuals from Portugal's continental region provided the ECG recordings used in this study. All volunteers in this study disclosed at least one previously diagnosed health condition, such as allergies, hypertension, cholesterol, diabetes, arrhythmia, asthma, unspecified heart problems, and unspecified brain problems; the most frequently disclosed conditions are hypertension and diabetes. The patient spends 30 s sitting down and 30 s standing during the ECG recordings, which at least takes about 60 s. This procedure tries to emphasize the differences between individuals (gender) and allow a minimum effort to avoid a significant change in the overall ECG result. Ethics Committee from Universidade da Beira Interior approved the study with the number CE-UBI-Pj-2021-41.

2.2 Feature Extraction

The NeuroKit Python module [29] was used to automatically extract important features from the ECG recordings for this study (Fig. 1), including P, Q, R, S, and T peaks, as well as the onsets and offsets of P, T, and R waves. Based on the features that were automatically retrieved and used in this investigation, the following features were manually calculated:

- RR interval $\rightarrow PeakR_N - PeakR_{N-1}$
- PP interval $\rightarrow PeakP_N - PeakP_{N-1}$
- P duration $\rightarrow OffsetP - OnsetP$
- PR interval $\rightarrow OnsetR - OnsetP$
- PR segment $\rightarrow OnsetR - OffsetP$

- QRS duration → $OffsetR - OnsetR$
- ST segment → $OnsetT - OffsetR$
- ST-T segment → $OffsetT - OffsetR$
- QT duration → $OffsetT - OnsetR$
- TP interval → $OnsetP - OffsetT$
- R amplitude → $PeakR_N - PeakS_N$
- T amplitude → $PeakT_N - PeakS_N$
- P amplitude → $PeakP_N - PeakQ_N$

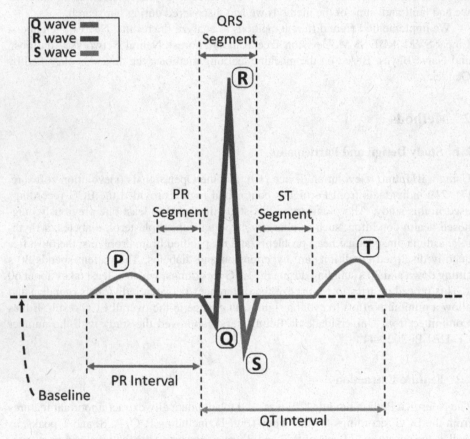

Fig. 1. Features from the ECG recordings

2.3 Description of the Method

We have implemented eight machine learning methods to analyze the results in the dataset that can predict some results.

Nearest Neighbors. K-Nearest Neighbors (K-NN) is a non-parametric technique that uses data from many classes to predict how the new sample point will be classified [26]. This algorithm does not use the training data points to draw any conclusions.

Linear SVM. The Support Vector Machine attempts to generate the best line or decision boundary to divide n-dimensional space into classes, so new data points are assigned to the correct category when added [5]. Support vectors are the extreme points/vectors that help this algorithm generate the best decision boundary and give the method its name [5]. The term linear SVM refers to linearly separable data, which can be divided into two classes using a single straight line [25].

RBF SVM. The Radial Basis Function (RBF) is the default kernel function in many kernelized learning algorithms [21]. It's very similar to the K-Nearest Neighborhood Algorithm, but instead of storing the entire dataset during training, the RBF SVM only needs to store the support vectors [12]. Linear SVM differs from RBF SVM in that the latter is not a parametric model like linear SVM, is more complex depending on the size of the database, and is more expensive to train [16].

Decision Tree. It is a rule-based supervised machine learning classifier that generates questions based on dataset properties and may categorize new entries depending on the answers [4]. It is a tree-based method because every question it creates has a binary response, which divides the database into halves [9]. A tree-like graph may be seen as the result of these divisions [9].

Random Forest. It is a machine learning algorithm widely applied to classification and regression issues [1]. It works by building decision trees on various samples throughout the training phase [1]. The outcome is determined based on the class with the most tree selections.

Neural Networks. It is commonly a multilayer perceptron with three layers: an input, a hidden layer, and an output layer [13, 15]. The last two layers are made up of nodes that function as neurons and make use of a nonlinear activation function. A multilayer perceptron can categorize data that is not linearly separable and uses backpropagation for training [22].

AdaBoost. It is an ensemble learning method that combines the results of various classifier algorithms to increase their effectiveness and predictive ability [14]. The output of the AdaBoost meta-algorithm is the outcome of this weighted sum.

Naive Bayes. Based on the Bayes theorem, it is a probabilistic machine learning method classifier [23, 28]. Its simplicity and lack of a complex iterative parameter calculation make it suitable for diagnosing cardiac patients in medical science [8]. This algorithm performs well and is popular because it frequently outperforms the most advanced classification techniques.

3 Results

3.1 Data Acquisition

For this study, we collected data from 219 volunteers (112 men, 106 women, and one other) aged between 12 and 92 years old. All participants provided informed consent to the experiments, allowing us to share the results anonymously. The agreement also provided informed consent to the participants regarding the risks and purpose of the study. Ethics Committee from Universidade da Beira Interior approved the study with the number CE-UBI-Pj-2021-041. The dataset used in this research is publicly available at [17].

Data were acquired with the BITalino (r)evolution device with a 1 kHz sample frequency, connected to a personal computer, using OpenSignals (r)evolution software. Each volunteer's data was stored in two files: one JSON file referring to the characteristic data of the volunteer plus their lifestyle and a text file with the test data recorded over time. These files were stored in an individual folder per volunteer.

The volunteer needed to stand for 30 s and then sit in a chair for 30 s while the data was collected.

The dataset is available in a Mendeley Data repository, which contains two files for each individual, with 219 folders. Each folder has a JSON file containing a description of the data acquisition conditions, the individual's characteristics, and the sensors used, and a TXT text file including the data acquired from the ECG sensor.

The Fig. 2 flowchart illustrates the data processing till the classification results.

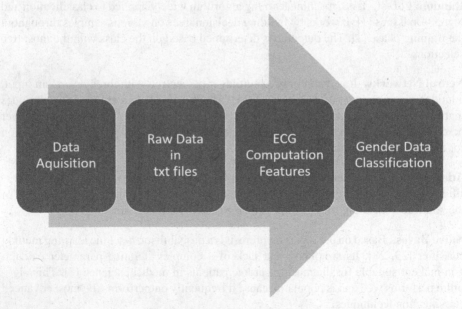

Fig. 2. Data processing flowchart

3.2 Results by Gender

We started with the extraction of the different analyzed variables related to the ECG data, such as RR interval, PP interval, P duration, PR interval, PR segment, QRS duration, ST segment, ST-T segment, QT duration, TP interval, R amplitude, T amplitude, and P amplitude. Table 1 presents the average of the features extracted. Before the analysis by gender, we found that the data of the individuals with the IDs 20, 25, 31, 33, 35, 38, 39, 54, 153, 195, and 202 were invalid, so it was necessary to exclude these 11 individuals from the analysis.

Table 1. Average of features extracted.

Features	Average
RR interval (ms)	856.76
PP interval (ms)	856.78
P duration (ms)	40.29
PR interval (ms)	123.98
PR segment interval (ms)	114.76
QRS duration (ms)	113.79
ST segment interval	157.25
ST-T segment interval (ms)	220.70
QT duration (ms)	334.49
TP interval (ms)	497.07
R amplitude (mV)	340.89
T amplitude (mV)	106.52
P amplitude (mV)	80.34

In Table 2, we compare the results of each classifier utilized during this study. The Decision Tree algorithm achieved the highest accuracy at 62.90%. Linear SVM, Adaboost, and Naive Bayes are right next, with an accuracy of 61.29%

Nearest Neighbors method correctly identified 32 male and female out of 62 volunteers in this study. It achieved an accuracy of 51.61%, a precision of 51.51%, a recall of 54.84%, and an F1-score of 53.14%. More details of this method are in the confusion matrix presented in Table 3.

As seen in Table 3, the Linear SVM classifier correctly identified 38 males and females out of 62, making it one of the methods that identified the highest numbers. This algorithm reached an accuracy of 61.29%, a precision of 51.72%, a recall of 78.13%, and an F1-score of 62.24%.

Table 2. Performance comparison of the various methods

Features	Accuracy (%)	Precision (%)	Recall (%)	F1-Score (%)
K-NN	51.61	51.51	54.84	53.14
Linear SVM	61.29	51.72	78.13	62.24
RBF SVM	48.38	38.46	16.67	23.26
Decision Tree	62.90	61.29	63.33	62.29
Random Forest	56.45	57.69	48.39	52.63
Neural Net	51.61	45.16	51.85	48.27
AdaBoost	61.29	46.67	63.63	53.85
Naive Bayes	61.29	46.67	63.63	53.85

From the ECG recordings in our dataset, the RBF SVM method was capable, as seen in Table 3, of accurately predicting 28 males and females. It achieved the lowest accuracy out of any method at 48.38%, a precision of 38.46%, a recall of 16.67%, and an F1-score of 23.26%.

The Decision Tree algorithm could identify the correct gender in 4 instances. As seen in Table 3, it correctly classified 19 of the recordings as belonging to males and 20 of them as belonging to a female. Overall, this method was the one that could have the highest percentages. It achieved an accuracy of 62.90%, a precision of 61.29%, a recall of 63.33%, and an F1-score of 62.29%.

The Random Forest classifier correctly predicted 35 results. As seen in Table 3, it identified 15 males and 20 females. This method reached an accuracy of 56.45%, a precision of 57.69%, a recall of 48.39%, and an F1-score of 52.63%.

As seen in Table 3, the Neural Network classifier utilized in this study correctly identified 14 males and 18 females, counting 32. This method reached an accuracy of 51.61%, a precision of 45.16%, a recall of 51.85%, and an F1-score of 48.27%.

As seen in Table 3, the AdaBoost algorithm correctly classified 38 of the 62 volunteers. It achieved an accuracy of 61.29%, a precision of 46.67%, a recall of 63.63%, and an F1-score of 53.85%.

The Decision Tree algorithm presented in Table 3 could identify the gender achieving 38 males and females out of 62 volunteers. Overall, it achieved an accuracy of 61.29%, a precision of 46.67%, a recall of 63.63%, and an F1-score of 53.85%.

Table 3. Confusion matrix for the results by gender

	Gender	TP	TN	FP	FN
K-NN	Male	17	15	16	14
	Female	15	17	14	16
Linear SVM	Male	25	13	17	7
	Female	13	25	7	17
RBF SVM	Male	5	23	8	25
	Female	23	5	25	8
Decision Tree	Male	19	20	12	11
	Female	20	19	11	12
Random Forest	Male	15	20	11	16
	Female	20	15	16	11
Neural Net	Male	14	18	17	13
	Female	18	14	13	17
AdaBoost	Male	14	24	16	8
	Female	24	14	8	16
Naive Bayes	Male	14	24	16	8
	Female	24	14	8	16

4 Discussions and Conclusions

We tested 8 methods on a dataset of ECG recordings to see how well they could categorize the data. We could use the confusion matrix produced by the application to our dataset to calculate each of these eight methods' accuracy, precision, recall, and F1-score. The Decision tree attained the best accuracy at 62.90%, followed by the Linear SVM, AdaBoost, and Naive Bayes approach at 61.29% of accuracy.

With these outcomes, we concluded that Decision Trees was the technique that performed the best overall, which accurately identified 39 of the 62 results. Our initial expectations met the outcomes of this investigation, as the best-performing approach could accurately classify more than 50% of males and females in these ECG recordings.

This study used a small database, which could influence the results presented in these studies. We expect to get more data to consolidate the results in the future.

Acknowledgments. This work is funded by FCT/MEC through national funds and co-funded by FEDER – PT2020 partnership agreement under the project **UIDB/50008/2020** (*Este trabalho é financiado pela FCT/MEC através de fundos nacionais e cofinanciado pelo FEDER, no âmbito do Acordo de Parceria PT2020 no âmbito do projeto UIDB/50008/2020*).

This article is based upon work from COST Action CA19136 - International Interdisciplinary Network on Smart Healthy Age-friendly Environments (NET4AGE-FRIENDLY), supported by COST (European Cooperation in Science and Technology). More information in www.cost.eu.

References

1. Alazzam, H., Alsmady, A., Shorman, A.A.: Supervised detection of IoT botnet attacks. In: Proceedings of the Second International Conference on Data Science, E-Learning and Information Systems, pp. 1–6 (2019)
2. AlDuwaile, D.A., Islam, M.S.: Using convolutional neural network and a single heartbeat for ECG biometric recognition. Entropy **23**, 733 (2021)
3. Ali, F., et al.: A smart healthcare monitoring system for heart disease prediction based on ensemble deep learning and feature fusion. Inf. Fus. **63**, 208–222 (2020)
4. Almuhaideb, S., Menai, M.E.B.: Impact of preprocessing on medical data classification. Front. Comput. Sci. **10**(6), 1082–1102 (2016). https://doi.org/10.1007/s11704-016-5203-5
5. Amarappa, S., Sathyanarayana, S.V.: Data classification using support vector machine (SVM), a simplified approach. Int. J. Electron. Comput. Sci. Eng. **3**, 435–445 (2014)
6. Balakumar, P., Maung-U, K., Jagadeesh, G.: Prevalence and prevention of cardiovascular disease and diabetes mellitus. Pharmacol. Res. **113**, 600–609 (2016)
7. Batista, D., Plácido da Silva, H., Fred, A., Moreira, C., Reis, M., Ferreira, H.A.: Benchmarking of the BITalino biomedical toolkit against an established gold standard. Healthc. Technol. Lett. **6**, 32–36 (2019)
8. Celin, S., Vasanth, K.: ECG signal classification using various machine learning techniques. J. Med. Syst. **42**, 1–11 (2018)
9. Chio, C., Freeman, D.: Machine Learning and Security: Protecting Systems With data and Algorithms. O'Reilly Media, Inc. (2018)
10. Da Silva, H.P., Guerreiro, J., Lourenço, A., Fred, A.L., Martins, R.: BITalino: a novel hardware framework for physiological computing. In: PhyCS, pp. 246–253 (2014)
11. Escobar, L.J.V., Salinas, S.A.: e-Health prototype system for cardiac telemonitoring. In: 2016 38th Annual International Conference of the IEEE Engineering in Medicine and Biology Society (EMBC), Orlando, FL, USA, pp. 4399–4402. IEEE (2016)
12. García, V., Mollineda, R.A., Sánchez, J.S.: On the k-NN performance in a challenging scenario of imbalance and overlapping. Pattern Anal. Appl. **11**, 269–280 (2008)
13. Gautam, M.K., Giri, V.K.: A neural network approach and wavelet analysis for ECG classification. In: 2016 IEEE International Conference on Engineering and Technology (ICETECH), Coimbatore, India, pp. 1136–1141. IEEE (2016)
14. Hastie, T., Rosset, S., Zhu, J., Zou, H.: Multi-class AdaBoost. Stat. Interface **2**, 349–360 (2009). https://doi.org/10.4310/SII.2009.v2.n3.a8
15. Haykin, S.: Neural Networks: A Comprehensive Foundation, 1st edn. Prentice Hall PTR, Hoboken (1994)
16. Hsu, C.-W., Lin, C.-J.: A comparison of methods for multiclass support vector machines. IEEE Trans. Neural Netw. **13**, 415–425 (2002)
17. Pires, I.M., Garcia, N.M., Pires, I., Pinto, R., Silva, P.: ECG data related to 30-s seated and 30-s standing for 5P-Medicine project. Mendeley Data (2022). https://data.mendeley.com/datasets/z4bbj9rcwd/1
18. Jindal, H., Agrawal, S., Khera, R., Jain, R., Nagrath, P.: Heart disease prediction using machine learning algorithms. In: IOP Conference Series: Materials Science and Engineering. IOP Publishing, p. 012072 (2021)
19. Kakria, P., Tripathi, N.K., Kitipawang, P.: A real-time health monitoring system for remote cardiac patients using smartphone and wearable sensors. Int. J. Telemed. Appl., 1–11 (2015). https://doi.org/10.1155/2015/373474
20. Kannathal, N., Acharya, U.R., Ng, E.Y.K., Krishnan, S.M., Min, L.C., Laxminarayan, S.: Cardiac health diagnosis using data fusion of cardiovascular and haemodynamic signals. Comput. Methods Programs Biomed. **82**, 87–96 (2006). https://doi.org/10.1016/j.cmpb.2006.01.009

21. Maji, S., Berg, A.C., Malik, J.: Classification using intersection kernel support vector machines is efficient. In: 2008 IEEE Conference on Computer Vision and Pattern Recognition, pp. 1–8. IEEE (2008)
22. Pires, I.M., Garcia, N.M., Flórez-Revuelta, F.: Multi-sensor data fusion techniques for the identification of activities of daily living using mobile devices. In: Proceedings of the ECMLPKDD (2015)
23. Prescott, G.J., Garthwaite, P.H.: A simple Bayesian analysis of misclassified binary data with a validation substudy. Biometrics **58**, 454–458 (2002)
24. Ramaraj, E.: A novel deep learning based gated recurrent unit with extreme learning machine for electrocardiogram (ECG) signal recognition. Biomed. Signal Process. Control **68**, 102779 (2021)
25. Suthaharan, S.: Support vector machine. In: Suthaharan, S. (ed.) Machine Learning Models and Algorithms for Big Data Classification. Integrated Series in Information Systems, vol. 36, pp. 207–235. Springer, Boston (2016). https://doi.org/10.1007/978-1-4899-7641-3_9
26. Tran, T.M., Le, X.-M.T., Nguyen, H.T., Huynh, V.-N.: A novel non-parametric method for time series classification based on k-nearest neighbors and dynamic time warping barycenter averaging. Eng. Appl. Artif. Intell. **78**, 173–185 (2019)
27. Vogel, B., et al.: The Lancet women and cardiovascular disease commission: reducing the global burden by 2030. Lancet **397**, 2385–2438 (2021)
28. Webb, G.I., Boughton, J.R., Wang, Z.: Not so Naive Bayes: aggregating one-dependence estimators. Mach. Learn. **58**, 5–24 (2005). https://doi.org/10.1007/s10994-005-4258-6
29. Neurophysiological Data Analysis with NeuroKit2 — NeuroKit2 0.2.1 documentation. https://neuropsychology.github.io/NeuroKit/. Accessed 10 July 2022

Exploiting Blood Volume Pulse and Skin Conductance for Driver Drowsiness Detection

Angelica Poli[1], Andrea Amidei[2], Simone Benatti[2], Grazia Iadarola[1], Federico Tramarin[2], Luigi Rovati[2], Paolo Pavan[2], and Susanna Spinsante[1(✉)]

[1] Department of Information Engineering, Polytechnic University of Marche, Ancona 60121, Italy
{a.poli,g.iadarola,s.spinsante}@staff.univpm.it
[2] Department of Engineering "E. Ferrari", University of Modena and Reggio Emilia, Modena 41125, Italy
{andrea.amidei,simone.benatti,federico.tramarin,luigi.rovati, paolo.pavan}@unimore.it

Abstract. Attention loss caused by driver drowsiness is a major risk factor for car accidents. A large number of studies are conducted to reduce the risk of car crashes, especially to evaluate the driver behavior associated to drowsiness state. However, a minimally-invasive and comfortable system to quickly recognize the physiological state and alert the driver is still missing. This study describes an approach based on Machine Learning (ML) to detect driver drowsiness through an Internet of Things (IoT) enabled wrist-worn device, by analyzing Blood Volume Pulse (BVP) and Skin Conductance (SC) signals. Different ML algorithms are tested on signals collected from 9 subjects to classify the drowsiness status, considering different data segmentation options. Results show that using a different window length for data segmentation does not influence ML performance.

Keywords: Internet of Things · Machine Learning · Wearable devices · Blood volume pulse · Skin conductance · Driver monitoring · Drowsiness detection

1 Introduction

Based on the World Health Organization estimates, car accidents are responsible for nearly 1.35 million deaths each year [1], primarily due to driver drowsiness [2].

Authors from Polytechnic University of Marche acknowledge the partial support provided by Marche Region in implementation of the financial programme POR MARCHE FESR 2014-2020, project "*Miracle*" (Marche Innovation and Research facilities for Connected and Sustainable Living Environments), CUP B28I19000330007, and the partial support by the financial program DM MiSE 5 Marzo 2018, project "*ChAALenge*"— F/180016/01-05/X43.

S. Spinsante et al. (Eds.): HealthyIoT 2022, LNICST 456, pp. 50–61, 2023.
https://doi.org/10.1007/978-3-031-28663-6_5

For this reason several research studies are aimed at detecting a driver's drowsiness, through the use of proper sensors joined with Machine Learning (ML) and Artificial Intelligence (AI) algorithms. In some cases, safety technologies exploiting on-board sensors are already implemented in cars, to classify the driving behavior by monitoring lane deviations combined with steering wheel rotation, and enriched by additional sensors, such as camera-based systems, capturing the driver's status. However, these systems aim to detect explicit signs of microsleeps or sleepy behavior (such as changes in visual facial descriptors, like estimated distance between the nose and mouth; blinks and longer closures; eye gaze location; face orientation), not drowsiness, that occurs with decreasing levels of arousal which vary by individual [3]. Stress, fatigue, and illness contribute to drowsiness, that declines the driver's cognitive capabilities, increasing the risk of accidents [4]. Moreover, the above-mentioned approaches exhibit some degrees of reliability but also suffer limitations due to uncontrollable operational conditions: variable lighting scenarios, or glasses and sunglasses worn by the driver may impact the expected detection capability. Different and innovative solutions have been consequently investigated, to overcome the mentioned limits.

Drowsiness influences the driver's behavior and is associated with the Autonomic Nervous System (ANS) activity reflected by changes in physiological signals [2]. Specifically, the Blood Volume Pulse (BVP) signal refers to the total amount of blood circulating within the arteries, capillaries, veins, venules, and chambers of the heart, at any given time [5]. BVP leads to the estimation of Heart Rate Variability (HRV), a useful indicator for both fatigue and drowsiness conditions, according to the literature [6,7]. The Skin Conductance (SC) signal is usually exploited to detect changes in a subject's arousal: it varies because of sweat gland secretion, and it can be decomposed in a slowly varying component, known as Skin Conductance Level (SCL) [8], plus a second component, featuring rapid changes in signal amplitude, known as Skin Conductance Response (SCR) [9]. For both the referenced signals, gold-standard measurement methods foresee the use of electrodes in direct skin contact, and applied on specific positions. In the case of the SC signal, it should be preferably acquired on fingers, foot or hand palms, where sweat glands are mostly spread. Unfortunately, the necessary skin contact of the sensors to acquire SC or Photoplethysmography (PPG) signals [10] is a major shortcoming of approaches based on physiological measurements in the automotive environment, where the common driving conditions are not compatible with the mentioned optimal sensor positioning choices.

For this reason, and pushed by the growing trends of the IoT-enabled wearables market, several studies tested wrist-worn devices (or wrist-worn-like ones, such as bracelets [11] and double-rings [12]) to collect physiological data that is then processed by classification algorithms to monitor drivers and detect a drowsy status [4]. As an example, Lee et al. assessed the driving behavior by utilizing the built-in motion sensor of a smartwatch; with a Support Vector Machine (SVM) classifier, an accuracy of 98.15% was achieved [13]. In another work, the same authors used the accelerometer signal combined with the PPG signal and they obtained an accuracy of 95.80% [14]. Instead, Leng et al. used a wearable device able to measure both PPG and SC signals on the fingers. The implemented SVM model reaches an accuracy of 98.70% [15]. Similarly, Choi et al. developed a wrist-worn wearable device with PPG, SC, temperature, acceleration, and gyroscope sensors. The SVM is employed to distinguish the normal, stressed, and drowsy states with an accuracy of about 85.00%. However, in this case, an additional PPG signal is acquired on the ear for more robust feature extraction, thus resulting in an intrusive system, less suitable for real-life driving applications [16]. In [17], we exploited the SC signal alone to assess driver's drowsiness, obtaining an accuracy equal to 84.1%. Later on, Li et al. [18] showed that a properly designed feature extracted from the SC signal could be used in driver's status management, and takeover-safety prediction for autonomous driving systems.

Wrist-worn devices represent an appealing solution for driver's monitoring since they allow physiological signal acquisition in a minimally invasive fashion, and future car implementations could directly interact with them, for a feasible and integrated approach to the driver's drowsiness detection problem. The device used in this work is the Empatica E4 wristband, which obtained CE medical certification in Europe, for acquired signals of better quality than the ones obtained from prototype devices, like those designed on purpose and used in other research works [15].

The analysis of recent literature shows that almost all the published works exploit ML or Deep Learning (DL) algorithms to process the data acquired from wearables and automatically classify the driver's condition. As such, it is reasonable to investigate if the way the collected data is pre-processed may affect the attainable classification accuracy. In this respect, the research presented in this paper exploits a minimally-invasive wrist-worn device to collect both BVP and SC physiological signals, with the aim to explore the ANS activity related to changes in the driver's arousal, which may be associated to a drowsy behavior. The collected time series of physiological data are pre-processed according to different sizes of data segmentation, before computing features used to feed three different ML algorithms to detect and classify driver's drowsiness. Based on the attained classification accuracy, the impact of the different data segment sizes chosen is investigated.

The paper is structured as follows: Sect. 2 describes the experimental setup and the acquisition protocol. Section 3 presents the performed data processing, while in Sect. 4 the obtained results are provided. Lastly, Sect. 5 draws the main conclusions and outlines possible future works.

2   Materials and Methods

2.1   Experimental Setup and Acquisition Device

For the purpose of this study, a driving simulator was placed in a room with an average ambient temperature of around 23°C. Temperature was maintained quite stable to reduce its influence on the user's skin (e.g., sweat or cold body), and consequently on physiological signals acquired during the experimental tests.

The route shown on the driving simulator was an overnight 80 km long driving path on a three-lane highway. A picture of the whole experimental setup is shown in Fig. 1.

During the driving simulation, and with the aim to propose an as much realistic as possible approach, BVP and SC signals were collected by wearing a single smart-band, the Empatica E4 [19], on the driver's dominant wrist. The E4 is a multi-sensor wrist-worn device able to detect changes in both user's cardiac activity and skin conductance, through two specific embedded sensors: PPG and SC sensor, respectively. By using a proprietary algorithm, the PPG sensor, equipped with 2 green LEDs and 2 red LEDs, extracts the BVP signal from the pulse waves at a fixed sampling rate 64 Hz. Regarding the SC, a small alternating current (maximum peak-to-peak value of 100 μA - at a frequency 8 Hz) moves through two Ag/AgCl electrodes located on the bottom side of the bracelet, and the electric skin conductance across the skin is acquired at a sampling frequency 4 Hz, a resolution of 900 pS, and a dynamic range of [0.01, 100] μS. Once an acquisition session terminates, data collected from all the sensors embedded into the E4 are stored into the Empatica Cloud, from which they can be downloaded for further post-processing and analysis.

2.2 Data Acquisition Protocol

Nine healthy subjects, namely five women and four men, were recruited for the test procedure. Since physiological data vary with age and gender, drivers have been chosen to cover the [28] years age range, that represents the age range of the majority of active drivers' population. Moreover, to avoid bias due to gender, we selected a male and a female driver in each age cohort of 10 years, from 20 to 60 years of age. After receiving information about the study, the participants signed the informed consent. Then, they were provided with the Empatica E4 device to be worn on the dominant wrist during the six simulated driving sessions (around 40 min-long each) to acquire simultaneously the BVP and SC signals. Samples of the acquired BVP and SC signals over a whole 40 min-long session are given in Fig. 2.

Every 10 min, the participants reported their own perceived level of drowsiness on a tablet, according to the 9-point Karolinska Sleepiness Scale (KSS) questionnaire [20]. Similarly to other studies [21], we used the KSS self-assessment measure to subjectively quantify the level of drowsiness of the participants.

3 Data Processing

The quality of signals acquired from the wrist, and consequently the performance of the driver's drowsiness detection, can be highly affected by natural body movements performed while driving. To identify and reduce the motion artifacts in SC signals [22], the Stationary Wavelet Transform (SWT) denoising with Haar mother wavelet (7 levels of decomposition) was implemented, according to previous studies [23]. This approach firstly models the wavelet coefficients by using

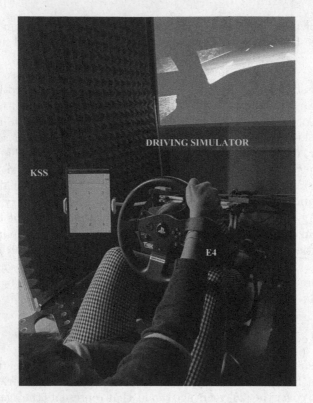

Fig. 1. The experimental setup used for acquisitions, including: the driving simulator, the tablet showing the KSS to select, and the E4 worn by the subject during tests.

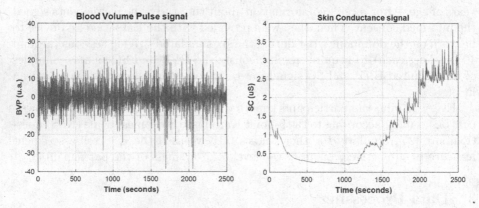

Fig. 2. Sample acquired BVP (left) and SC (right) signals during a whole session (40 min duration).

zero-mean Laplace distribution, then it defines high and low thresholds to distinguish clean SC signal and motion artifacts. When the wavelet coefficients exceed these thresholds, they are set to zero. Then, the application of SWT results in a denoised signal. Regarding the BVP signal, an algorithm embedded in Empatica E4 firmware (the details of which are not disclosed by the manufacturer) removes the motion artifacts, by exploiting the signal measured during exposure to the red LED. Being the HRV a well-known drowsiness indicator [24], it was derived from the BVP signal, by quantifying the inter-beat intervals (i.e., the distance between two consecutive signal peaks). The obtained HRV and SC signals (both SCR and SCL components) were divided into time intervals with a fixed size of Δt seconds, and an overlapping window of length $\Delta t/2$ s. It is explained later on in the paper that different Δt values have been tested.

According to the 9-point KSS scale scores reported by the participants, each data window was labeled to detect the associated drowsiness status. Specifically, the KSS responses were grouped into two classes depending on the selected drowsiness level: KSS scores lower or equal to 6 (from 1 to 6) in class 1 (labeled as awake), and scores greater than 6 (from 7 to 9) in class 2 (labeled as drowsy). Finally, a total of 32 features, chosen in both time and frequency domains as listed in Table 1, was computed for each window. The features were considered in some cases since already used in previous studies [25–27], or, in other cases, such as the SC peaks, since characterized by a significant information content [28,29].

As a first choice, $\Delta t = 30$ s and an overlapping of 15 s were considered [25,30]. Such a window size was chosen according to [30], in which authors state that drowsiness can be detected in short periods. Then to study the effect of the time window length on the performance of the ML classifiers tested, the analysis was repeated by considering different sizes of data segmentation. In particular, segmentation windows with a length of 15 s, 45 s, and 60 s, were considered, and a 50% overlap, to preserve the condition applied in the first analysis.

Table 1. Features extracted from HRV and SC.

Type of signal	Domain	Features
HRV signal	Time	HR (bpm), SDNN (ms), RMSSD (a.u.), pNN50 (μS)
	Frequency	LF (a.u./Hz), HF (a.u./Hz), LFn (a.u./Hz), HFn (a.u./Hz), LF/HF (a.u.)
SC signal	Time	Mean (μS), standard deviation (μS), minimum (μS), maximum (μS), kurtosis (μS), skewness (μS), variance (($\mu S)^2$), range (μS), median (μS)
	Frequency	Mean (μS/Hz), standard deviation (μS/Hz), minimum (μS/Hz), maximum (μS/Hz), kurtosis (μS/Hz), skewness (μS/Hz), variance ((μS/Hz)^2), range (μS/Hz), median (μS/Hz)
SC components	Time	SCR number of peaks, SCL mean (μS), SCL standard deviation (μS), SCL minimum (μS), SCL maximum (μS)

56   A. Poli et al.

Following the two steps of data pre-processing and feature extraction, several ML algorithms were tested in MATLAB by means of the Classification Learner Toolbox. All the features were considered with a 10-fold cross-validation on input data. For each window, to perform ML analysis, the dataset was divided randomly into training and testing sets, corresponding, respectively, to 80% and 20% of the entire set. Since at each run of the classifiers the two groups are different, we tested every algorithm 10 times for all size windows, then we calculated the mean value of the obtained classification accuracy. To improve ML performance, features were normalized by their maximum value in each window, resulting in the range [0, 1]. Data analysis and feature extraction were performed in MATLAB environment. Figure 3 summarizes the different steps of the applied data processing.

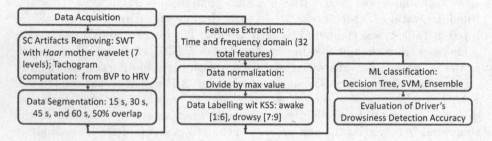

Fig. 3. Graphical summary of the applied processing steps.

Table 2. Accuracy of different classifiers with the tested approaches.

Classifier	Accuracy (%)	Windows length (s)
Decision Tree	83.5	15
SVM	88.3	
Ensemble	93.0	
Decision Tree	83.2	30
SVM	89.2	
Ensemble	92.2	
Decision Tree	83.5	45
SVM	88.8	
Ensemble	91.8	
Decision Tree	84.7	60
SVM	90.0	
Ensemble	91.1	

4   Results

The classification performance was assessed based on the accuracy provided by each algorithm, and obtained by considering different lengths of the time windows applied for data segmentation. The accuracy provided by a classification algorithm is defined as:

$$Accuracy = (1 - ErrorRate) \cdot 100 \qquad (1)$$

where $ErrorRate = -N_{cci} \cdot N_{ti} - /N_{ti}$, being N_{cci} and N_{ti} the numbers of correctly classified instances and total instances, respectively.

The length of the time windows used to evaluate and compare the classification performance are summarized in Table 2. The tested algorithms with the highest performance are Decision Tree, SVM, and Ensemble. Considering the 30 s-long window, i.e. the first tested window length, the best result was achieved by Ensemble with an accuracy of 92.2%, then SVM with 89.3%, and Decision Tree with 83.2%. However, taking into account all the analyzed window lengths, the best results were achieved by Ensemble considering a 15 s-long window with an accuracy of 93.0%. SVM and Decision Tree reached the highest performance with an accuracy of 90.0% and 84.7% respectively, both considering a window of 60 s. The results are comparable to the previously discussed works [13–16].

Figure 4 shows the results in terms of accuracy for different lengths of acquisition time windows. It is clear there are no significant differences among all the considered values, demonstrating that the physiological onset of drowsiness conditions is a slow phenomenon. Additionally, high accuracy levels and slight performance variations make the obtained results more robust since they confirm that it is possible to obtain a high classification accuracy value, even considering several lengths of the time windows.

The results herein presented, obtained on a dataset including few subjects, suggest the possibility to detect, by proper classifiers, the drowsiness condition in drivers. High classification accuracy has been obtained by considering signals collected from a minimally invasive wrist-worn device, which may represent an important outcome towards practical solutions to the problem of increasing drivers' safety.

58   A. Poli et al.

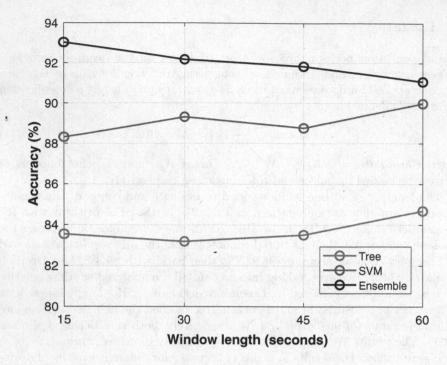

Fig. 4. ML accuracy of the tested algorithms considering different time windows. The black line refers to the Ensemble classifier, the blue line to SVM, the red line to the Decision Tree algorithm. (Color figure online)

5 Conclusions and Future Works

This study focused on the detection of driver's drowsiness based on BVP and SC physiological variations, recorded through a wrist-worn device during a simulated overnight driving session. In particular, the authors attempted to classify the alert status from the drowsy one, by testing three ML algorithms. Since BVP and SC signals are linked to ANS activity, 32 features were extracted from cited physiological signals. They were segmented in time windows of 15 s, 30 s, 45 s, and 60 s with an overlap interval equal to 50% of the considered window length. Although the dataset is limited, it covers a wide range of ages (28–60 years) and it is also gender-balanced since drivers are 4 males and 5 females. Table 2 and Fig. 4 prove that the drowsiness detection capability of the tested classifiers is not affected by the choice of the window length used for data segmentation. In fact, using a shorter window length value instead of a longer one does not change significantly the attainable accuracy. For two classifiers out of three (namely, Decision Tree and SVM), increasing the window length slightly improves the classification accuracy: this could support the idea that drowsiness onset is a slow process, better detected on a longer observation time. In the end, we can say the obtained results demonstrate the possibility to detect drivers' drowsiness reliably.

In future works, we will perform driving tests on a larger number of drivers with the purpose to involve drivers in the age range between 18 and 28 years, as well as in the range of 60–80 years age. This way, we will test a population including almost all the ages for which a driving license is allowed. We will study ML performance considering larger windows for data segmentation (i.e. 1 min, 2 min, 5 min) to investigate the rapidity of drowsiness level variation. Also, we will investigate the effects of features normalization on the classifiers to find the best data processing approach for drivers' drowsiness detection. Based on these studies, we will develop a custom algorithm to further improve detection accuracy.

References

1. WHO - Global Status Report on Road Safety 2018. https://www.who.int/publications/i/item/9789241565684
2. Khan, M.Q., Lee, S.: A comprehensive survey of driving monitoring and assistance systems. Sensors **19**, 2574 (2019). https://doi.org/10.3390/s19112574
3. Schwarz, C., Gaspar, J., Miller, T., Yousefian, R.: The detection of drowsiness using a driver monitoring system. Traffic Inj. Prev. **20**, S157–S161 (2019). https://doi.org/10.1080/15389588.2019.1622005
4. Saleem, A.A., Siddiqui, H.U.R., Raza, M.A.: A systematic review of physiological signals based driver drowsiness detection systems. Cogn. Neurodyn. (2022). https://doi.org/10.1007/s11571-022-09898-9
5. Convertino, V.A.: Blood volume: its adaptation to endurance training. Med. Sci. Sports Exerc. **23**, 1338–1348 (1991)
6. Kaplan, S., Guvensan, M.A., Yavuz, A.G., Karalurt, Y.: Driver behavior analysis for safe driving: a survey. IEEE Trans. Intell. Transp. Syst. **16**, 3017–3032 (2015). https://doi.org/10.1109/TITS.2015.2462084
7. Cosoli, G., Iadarola, G., Poli, A., Spinsante, S.: Learning classifiers for analysis of blood volume pulse signals in IoT-enabled systems. In: Proceedings of the 2021 IEEE International Workshop on Metrology for Industry 4.0 IoT (MetroInd4.0 IoT), pp. 307–312, June 2021
8. Iadarola, G., Poli, A., Spinsante, S.: Compressed sensing of skin conductance level for IoT-based wearable sensors. In: Proceedings of the 2022 IEEE International Instrumentation and Measurement Technology Conference (I2MTC), pp. 1–6 (2022)
9. Iadarola, G., Poli, A., Spinsante, S.: Reconstruction of galvanic skin response peaks via sparse representation. In: Proceedings of the 2021 IEEE International Instrumentation and Measurement Technology Conference (I2MTC), pp. 1–6 (2021)
10. Amidei, A., Fallica, P.G., Conoci, S., Pavan, P.: Validating Photoplethysmography (PPG) data for driver drowsiness detection. In: Proceedings of the 2021 IEEE International Workshop on Metrology for Automotive (MetroAutomotive), pp. 147–151, July 2021
11. STEER: Wearable Device That Will Not Let You Fall Asleep. https://www.kickstarter.com/projects/creativemode/steer-you-will-never-fall-asleep-while-driving. Accessed 13 May 2022
12. StopSleep: The Best Solution against Drowsiness. https://www.stopsleep.co.uk/. Accessed 13 May 2022

13. Lee, B.-L., Lee, B.-G., Chung, W.-Y.: Standalone wearable driver drowsiness detection system in a smartwatch. IEEE Sens. J. **16**, 5444–5451 (2016). https://doi.org/10.1109/JSEN.2016.2566667

14. Lee, B.-G., Lee, B.-L., Chung, W.-Y.: Smartwatch-based driver alertness monitoring with wearable motion and physiological sensor. In: Proceedings of the 2015 37th Annual International Conference of the IEEE Engineering in Medicine and Biology Society (EMBC), pp. 6126–6129, August 2015

15. Leng, L.B., Giin, L.B., Chung, W.-Y.: Wearable driver drowsiness detection system based on biomedical and motion sensors. In: Proceedings of the 2015 IEEE SENSORS, pp. 1–4, November 2015

16. Choi, M., Koo, G., Seo, M., Kim, S.W.: Wearable device-based system to monitor a driver's stress, fatigue, and drowsiness. IEEE Trans. Instrum. Meas. **67**, 634–645 (2018). https://doi.org/10.1109/TIM.2017.2779329

17. Amidei, A., et al.: Driver drowsiness detection based on variation of skin conductance from wearable device. In: IEEE International Workshop on Metrology for Automotive (2022)

18. Li, P., Li, Y., Yao, Y., Wu, C., Nie, B., Li, S.E.: Sensitivity of electrodermal activity features for driver arousal measurement in cognitive load: the application in automated driving systems. IEEE Trans. Intell. Transp. Syst. **23**(9), 14954–14967 (2022). https://doi.org/10.1109/TITS.2021.3135266

19. E4 WristBand from Empatica User's Manual (2008)

20. Shahid, A., Wilkinson, K., Marcu, S., Shapiro, C.M.: Karolinska sleepiness scale (KSS). In: Shahid, A., Wilkinson, K., Marcu, S., Shapiro, C.M. (eds.) STOP, THAT and One Hundred Other Sleep Scales, pp. 209–210. Springer, New York (2011). https://doi.org/10.1007/978-1-4419-9893-4_47, ISBN 978-1-4419-9892-7

21. Dunbar, J., Gilbert, J.E., Lewis, B.: Exploring differences between self-report and electrophysiological indices of drowsy driving: a usability examination of a personal brain-computer interface device. J. Safety Res. **74**, 27–34 (2020). https://doi.org/10.1016/j.jsr.2020.04.006

22. Chen, W., Jaques, N., Taylor, S., Sano, A., Fedor, S., Picard, R.W.: Wavelet-Based Motion Artifact Removal for Electrodermal Activity. In: Annual International Conference of the IEEE Engineering in Medicine and Biology Society, IEEE Engineering in Medicine and Biology Society, Annual International Conference on 2015, pp. 6223–6226 (2015). https://doi.org/10.1109/EMBC.2015.7319814

23. Shukla, J., Barreda-Ángeles, M., Oliver, J., Puig, D.: Efficient wavelet-based artifact removal for electrodermal activity in real-world applications. Biomed. Signal Process. Control **42**, 45–52 (2018). https://doi.org/10.1016/j.bspc.2018.01.009

24. Iwamoto, H., Hori, K., Fujiwara, K., Kano, M.: Real-driving-implementable drowsy driving detection method using heart rate variability based on long short-term memory and autoencoder. IFAC-Papers On Line **54**(15), 526–531 (2021). https://doi.org/10.1016/j.ifacol.2021.10.310

25. Ryu, G., et al.: Flexible and printed PPG sensors for estimation of drowsiness. IEEE Trans. Electron. Dev. (2018). https://doi.org/10.1109/TED.2018.2833477

26. Can, Y.S., Gokay, D., Kılıç, D.R., Ekiz, D., Chalabianloo, N., Ersoy, C.: How laboratory experiments can be exploited for monitoring stress in the wild: a bridge between laboratory and daily life. Sensors **20**, 838 (2020). https://doi.org/10.3390/s20030838

27. Islam, A., Ma, J., Gedeon, T., Hossain, M.Z., Liu, Y.H.: Measuring user responses to driving simulators. In: 2nd IEEE International Conference on Artificial Intelligence and Virtual Reality, AIVR 2019. Proc. - 2019 IEEE International Conference Artificial Intelligent Virtual Real. AIVR 2019, pp. 33–40 (2019). https://doi.org/10.1109/AIVR46125.2019.00015
28. Iadarola, G., Poli, A., Spinsante, S.: Analysis of galvanic skin response to acoustic stimuli by wearable devices. In: Proceedings of the 2021 IEEE International Symposium on Medical Measurements and Applications (MeMeA), pp. 1–6, June 2021
29. Casaccia, F., Iadarola, G., Poli, A., Spinsante, S.: CS-based decomposition of acoustic stimuli-driven GSR peaks sensed by an IoT-enabled wearable device. In: Spinsante, S., Silva, B., Goleva, R. (eds.) HealthyIoT 2021. LNICST, vol. 432, pp. 166–179. Springer, Cham (2022). https://doi.org/10.1007/978-3-030-99197-5_14
30. Gwak, J., Shino, M., Early, H.A., Detection of driver drowsiness utilizing machine learning based on physiological signals, behavioral measures, and driving performance. In: 21st International Conference Intelligent Transport System ITSC **2018** (2018). https://doi.org/10.1109/ITSC.2018.8569493

Skin Conductance Under Acoustic Stimulation: Analysis by a Portable Device

Valeria Bruschi$^{(\boxtimes)}$ ⓘ, Nefeli Dourou ⓘ, Grazia Iadarola ⓘ, Angelica Poli ⓘ, Susanna Spinsante ⓘ, and Stefania Cecchi ⓘ

Department of Information Engineering, Polytechnic University of Marche, Ancona 60121, Italy
v.bruschi@pm.univpm.it, {n.a.dourou,g.iadarola, a.poli,s.spinsante,s.cecchi}@staff.univpm.it

Abstract. Skin Conductance (SC) variations, or, alternatively, changes of the human skin resistance known as Galvanic Skin Response (GSR), allow to detect the physiological reactions of a subject to different stimuli, either physical, or emotional and cognitive. This paper presents the analysis of SC variations under acoustic stimulation, performed by using a low-cost portable device designed for experimental use, able to acquire the human skin resistance values, which can be easily converted into SC ones. Preliminary findings, despite not generalizable because of the small set of participants involved in experiments, suggest that the reaction to sounds perceived as not pleasant is quite clear to identify, while further investigations are needed for acoustic stimuli classified as pleasant.

Keywords: Skin conductance · Acoustic stimulation · Portable device · Emotional state recognition

1 Introduction

In recent years, several hardware technologies and signal processing techniques have been developed to integrate different physiological measures into single portable or wearable devices, often enabled with wireless connectivity (according to the Internet of Things paradigm), with the aim of acquiring a broad range of parameters to evaluate different dimensions of an individual's status, from the physical and health-related ones [11,32], to the cognitive and emotional ones [7,9,24].

Among the signals of interest to collect, the Skin Conductance (SC), also known as Galvanic Skin Response (GSR) or Electrodermal Activity (EDA), plays

This work is partially supported by Marche Region in implementation of the financial programme POR MARCHE FESR 2014-2020, project *"Miracle"* (Marche Innovation and Research facilities for Connected and Sustainable Living Environments), CUP B28I19000330007, and partially supported by the financial program DM MiSE 5 Marzo 2018, project *"ChAALenge"*—F/180016/01-05/X43.

S. Spinsante et al. (Eds.): HealthyIoT 2022, LNICST 456, pp. 62–78, 2023.
https://doi.org/10.1007/978-3-031-28663-6_6

an important role, especially to investigate the relationship between physiological status and external stimuli, such as sensory, emotional, cognitive or physical ones [1,21,34]. The electrodermal activity reflects the changes in electrical conductance of the skin, which is modulated by sweat glands activity. An increase in sweating, mostly composed by water, increases the capability of the skin to conduct an electrical current. As all the eccrine sweat glands spread over the body skin are involved by emotion-evoked sweating, it is recognised that SC may provide a quantitative functional measure of the human symphatetic functions, such as cognitive or emotional arousal [17]. When a subject is exposed to some physical, emotional or cognitive events, the activity of the Autonomic Nervous System (ANS) affects the secretion of sweat glands, resulting in a variation of the EDA values [4].

Actually, the EDA signal consists of two main components, namely tonic and phasic levels. The tonic level, known as Skin Conductance Level (SCL), reflects slow changes in skin conductance, depending on skin dryness, hydration and automatic regulation. Instead, the phasic level or Skin Conductance Response (SCR) represents the dynamic changes associated to stimuli [4]. Hence, the SCRs induced by skin sweating are indicators of both psychological [5] and emotional status [38] of the considered individual.

Regarding the emotional status, acoustic stimulation is possible to induce emotional reaction and to affect physiological responses on humans. Three different types of audio stimuli are reported in the literature: (i) speech, (ii) music and (iii) general sounds, i.e., non-verbal and non-musical sounds [37]. In particular, music has the ability to regulate humans' emotions [25]; conversely, an individual's mood may affect preferences in music listening [12]. A possible mechanism behind the aforementioned regulation may be that music initiates brainstem responses, which successively modulate SC, as well heart rate, blood pressure, body temperature and muscle tension [6]. In addition to the brainstem responses, five more mechanisms, namely evaluative conditioning, emotional contagion, visual imaginary, episodic memory and musical expectancy are hypothesized to be involved in the musical induction of emotions [26]. The analysis of the above mechanisms is out of the scope of this work. As regards the humans' sense of hearing, the auditory nervous system is responsible for the conversion of the soundwave delivered at the entrance of the outer ear into information to the human brain. Sound reaches as soundwave (i.e., increase and increase of air molecules' pressure) at the entrance of the outer ear and, after passing the ear canal, it vibrates the tympanic membrane (i.e., transformed to mechanical energy). Following, within the cochlea, vibration is converted to electrical signal by the auditory hair cells, which in turn is delivered through the auditory nerve to the brainstem. [2,19].

As acoustic stimuli may elicit individuals' arousal, the acquisition of the corresponding EDA signals may support a quantitative evaluation of the generated effects. EDA signals may be collected in a so-called endosomatic fashion, meaning that no external source of electricity is used, or by an exosomatic approach, in which electrodes in direct contact with the skin allow to apply a constant current or voltage source. The second approach is far more common in wearable devices, as it does not require to collect the voltage between an active site and a relatively inactive one of the skin, despite the design of the corresponding acquisition device would be simpler in the former case. Using the exosomatic approach, the Ohm's law is exploited to compute the skin conductance (or conversely, its resistance) by measuring how the applied current or voltage is modulated by the electrodermal activity of the subject.

In this context, the aim of this work is to acquire SC signals through a portable low-cost device, and to analyse their variations under acoustic stimulation. The advantage of using a simple and low-cost portable device to collect SC signals relies in the possibility to run different types of experiments without the use of bulky equipment, and to have full control of the system settings [13]. Raw signal samples can be collected and processed by means of algorithms selected or designed on purpose, depending on the specific study targets [22]. In this work, the portable device was used to collect SC signals from six subjects, starting from their baseline EDA, then moving to the acquisition of their galvanic skin response as a result of different types of auditory stimulation, namely audio tracks of different genres. Acquisitions were performed out of laboratory settings, thus allowing a more realistic footprint of the subjects' reactions.

The paper is organized as follows. Section 2 describes the background studies on the effects of audio stimulation and on measurement devices for SC. Section 3 introduces the prototype components used for the experiments and explains the data collection procedure. Section 4 discusses the experimental results. Finally, Sect. 5 reports the conclusions.

2   Background

Many studies on the effects of the audio stimulation on human beings can be found in the literature. In particular, knowing how a particular audio stimulus can affect the listener is an important task for all the applications where a personalized listening experience is required. In [31], a genre-free model of five factors is introduced to classify the music preference of a subject in terms of emotional/affective responses. In [12,35], the audio equalization preference was investigated through subjective tests, that have proved the tendency of choosing a personalized equalization. In the last years, studies have aimed at finding a more objective evaluation of the perceived sound, comparing to the subjective self-reporting procedures. Furthermore, listening experience should be evaluated under real life, out-of-lab conditions and not through time-consuming, self-reporting, in-lab procedures. Thus, an alternative is the evaluation through physiological parameters measurements [29] collected by means of portable and easy-to-use devices.

In this context, the GSR signal has raised attention as a possible way to attain a more objective evaluation of the audio stimuli from the listeners' point of view, contrary to the mostly subjective self-reporting procedures. Additionally, a listener's GSR may be acquired during the process of auditory stimulation in a minimally invasive fashion, without interfering or interrupting the listening experience. This section reviews the works found in literature and related to GSR measurements under audio stimulation.

Several works aim at investigating the relationship between the GSR and the emotion induced on a listener by an audio stimuli. In recent works, the relationship between GSR and the pleasure induced on the listener [16, 20, 28], as well the arousal induced on the listener [16], considering the ground truth pleasure and arousal values taken by the IADS database [39], was investigated. In [36], the GSR measurement under music stimulation indicated that subjects not involved in music or not enjoying music gave little response of GSR. Moreover, GSR was used in [3] to measure the relaxation induced to individuals under the effect of binaural phenomena, in [30] to evaluate the effect of 3D sound on relaxation, and in [38] to test peoples' emotional responses to horror music. In [8], the effect of environmental noise on GSR was investigated. In [40], Zhang *et al.* presented the PMEmo dataset, which contains the perceived valence and arousal annotations of 794 songs along with the simultaneous GSR signals acquisitions. Except from the emotion, sound quality is another very important attribute to investigate. In fact, in [29], the correlation between the subjective assessment of perceived sound quality and the GSR was analyzed, however the meaningfulness of the specific physiological parameter for the sound quality evaluation was not able to be proven. Despite there is not, to the authors' best knowledge, a formal protocol for GSR acquisition under audio stimulation, it was observed that the aforementioned experimenters followed, some to a greater and others to a lesser extent, the following principles:

- The GSR of every participant is recorded during both, the presence and the absence (i.e., "baseline" period) of audio stimulation. Different factors (e.g., skin dryness, nervousness, temperature) result to different "baseline" GSR among participants [3]. Thus, the knowledge of GSR under no audio stimuli is necessary for calibrating the acquisitions of each participant under audio stimuli.
- Any external stimulation, besides the audio under examination, should be avoided during the GSR acquisition. Thus, GSR acquisition has been mostly conducted under in-lab conditions, to avoid any other undesirable cognitive process that could affect the GSR, and eyes are required to be closed to avoid any visual interference.
- The audio stimuli duration is not too long, to avoid the habituation phenomenon (i.e., the familiarization of the participant with the stimuli).
- The audio stimuli order presentation should be randomized to avoid the ordering effect.

2.1   Commercial Portable Devices for SC Acquisition

Looking at the commercial portable devices for SC-based monitoring found in the market, it is relevant to notice how there is not a huge variety of choices available, and most of them are quite expensive. The different options are presented in the following paragraphs.

The *Empatica E4* is a clinically validated device (Class IIa Medical Device according to 93/42/EEC Directive), equipped with four monitoring sensors, namely a 3-axes accelerometer, a photoplethysmography (PPG) sensor, an optical thermometer and an SC sensor. In particular, the SC sensor detects the electrical conductance across the skin by passing a very small alternating current (8 Hz frequency, 100 μA peak-to-peak amplitude) between two dry electrodes located on the bracelet, in contact with the bottom wrist. SC signals are collected at a sampling frequency 4 Hz, with a dynamic range of 0.01–100 μS and a resolution of 900 pS. The device may operate either in streaming and recording mode, and comes with a desktop application (E4 Manager) to transfer data to a cloud repository; a web application (E4 Connect) to visualize and manage data; a mobile application (E4 RealTime) to stream (via Bluetooth Low Energy) and visualize data in real-time, on mobile devices. Since a few months, the device has been discontinued by the manufacturer, so in the future it will be not available anymore for research studies. The device has been used in research studies, to measure the impact of auditory emotional stimuli [28], or to recognize the user emotions while watching short videos [41].

The *Empatica Embrace* is equipped with four sensors, namely a 3-axial accelerometer, a thermometer, a 3-axial gyroscope and an SC sensor. The last one detects the SC with a dynamic range of 0–80 μS and a resolution of 900 fS, at a sampling frequency 4 Hz. Specifically, three electrodes located on the bracelet and in contact with either the ventral (inner) and dorsal (outer) wrist are passed by an alternating current 4 Hz maximum frequency. Data are continuously sent via Bluetooth, and analysed in real-time to identify unusual patterns in movement and skin conductance. In fact, the smartband has been mainly involved in studies for seizure tracking and epilepsy management.

The *Gobe2* smart band is equipped with four embedded sensors, namely a bioimpedance sensor, an accelerometer, a piezo sensor and an SC sensor. For what concerns the individual's emotion, the *Gobe2* detects a so-called emotional tension, strictly associated with feelings and mood, by analysing the changes in cutaneous sweating. After evaluating these changes, the smart band notifies the users about their emotional status, with a vibration and a message on the display. The manufacturer declares that *GoBe* can detect the human stress, by using derived measurements, namely heart rate, previous night's sleep quality and personal details (i.e., weight, height, sex and age). A fully charged *GoBe2* can transfer data, through BLE, to a dedicated app and work for up to 48 h. No further details about the SC sensor are available, to the best of authors' knowledge.

The *Moodmetric* is a ring device specialised for measuring the SC: it collects SC levels and converts them into a scale ranging from 1 to 100, where higher values indicate higher arousal that can have either positive (e.g., excitement) or negative valence (e.g., stress). Approximately, the scores in the range 1–20 reflect a state of deep relaxation (e.g., meditational state); from 21 to 40, a regular

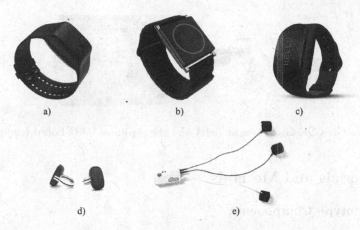

Fig. 1. SC-enabled portable devices available in the market: a) Empatica E4, b) Empatica Embrace, c) Gobe2, d) Moodmetric rings, e) Shimmer GSR+.

relaxation (e.g., walking); range 41–60 denotes mild activities (e.g., talking); 61–80, arousal during elevated activity (e.g., working under mild pressure); and 81–100, high arousal such as strong emotions. No details are available about the way these ranges are estimated from the raw data collected from the device, which is transferred by Bluetooth connection to a computer, for long term storage.

Finally, the *Shimmer3 GSR+* unit provides connections and pre-amplification for one channel of GSR data acquisition, and it is suitable for measuring the electrical characteristics or conductance of the skin, as well as jointly capturing an Optical Pulse/PPG signal to estimate heart rate, using the Shimmer ear clip or optical pulse probe. The collected samples are processed by a companion PC software, to compute different data features. The above mentioned devices are shown in Fig. 1.

As described above, specific algorithms for each device are able to process the collected raw data and provide the user with an output figure or index related to stress, or other conditions. Such processing typically takes place at the firmware level, or at the application level of a companion software, and related details are not available to users. This prevents the possibility to access the true signal samples, and to design or test different approaches to filtering or processing, e.g., for research purposes, as well as to evaluate precision and accuracy of the measured values. For this reason, it may be useful to setup a portable and low-cost device for SC that allows to collect unprocessed raw signal samples, for experimental usage.

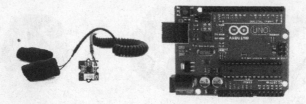

Fig. 2. The GSR-Grove sensor (left) and the Arduino UNO board (right).

3   Materials and Methods

3.1   Prototype Components

The prototype designed for the acquisition of the SC signal in this study is based on the Arduino UNO embedded platform, equipped with an ATmega328P microcontroller, and a GSR-Grove Sensor v1.2 [33], as shown in Fig. 2. The prototype collects samples of the skin resistance, thanks to two embedded Nickel electrodes worn in direct contact to the finger skin, applied through two small velcro bands. The GSR sensor operates at 3.3 V or 5 V, and its sensitivity may be adjusted via a potentiometer. A 4-wire cable is used to connect the GSR sensor to the Arduino UNO board. The signal acquired by the sensor is the skin resistance, encoded into an analogue voltage reading. To remove glitches, the code embedded into the firmware computes the average resistance value over 20 samples, in a 100 ms time interval. This way, resistance samples are acquired at a frequency 10 Hz. The analog skin resistance values are converted into 10-bit digital ones. It follows that the digital resistance values will range from a minimum of 0 to a maximum of 1023. By acting on the sensor potentiometer, the open circuit output (i.e., when the electrodes are not applied on fingers) may be set to 512, i.e., at the center of the output values range, to take advantage of the whole sensor dynamics. When using the device, power is preferably provided by an external supply, for better signal stability, and a USB cable connected to a PC allows to save data values into a file, for further processing.

3.2   Data Collection Protocol

In a first data collection session aimed at acquiring signals of relaxation state at rest condition, 2 young subjects (both 23 years old) were involved. Since fingers are among the most sensitive SC measurement sites and strongly respond to stimulation [27] (together with hand palms and foot soles) the sensor electrodes were placed on both index and middle fingers of the non-dominant hand with velcro stripes, as shown in Fig. 3. Following the open-circuit calibration of the device, the electrodes were suitably worn for ensuring the best adherence on the skin, and guaranteeing an accurate acquisition. As suggested in [23], prior to collecting data, the two individuals were instructed to breathe normally, keep limb movements to a minimum, try not to talk, and seat comfortably in a natural position. This procedure aimed to collect the subject's basal state and also to minimize artefacts.

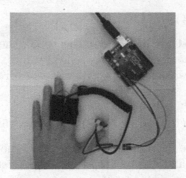

Fig. 3. Position of the wearable Arduino-based Grove GSR sensor.

GSR values were collected for 7 days, 3 times per day (i.e. after breakfast, after lunch, and after dinner) with a duration of 5 min per each acquisition. A total of 105 min of data, for each individual, was recorded in a week. Such data, acquired with the sampling frequency set 20 Hz, was transferred by directly connecting Arduino platform to a PC, saved in .txt files by using Coolterm software tool, and then analysed in Matlab environment.

Then, a data collection protocol was defined for experiments with acoustic stimulation. Six subjects, 5 females and 1 male, in the age range 20–51 years, were asked to lay supine on a bed, with arms at their sides, and to settle in a comfortable position. A bedroom was chosen as a recording environment, paying attention to have controlled ambient conditions to put the subjects at ease, and avoid light stimuli. Before connecting the equipment, some precautions were suggested to make the acquisitions more precise: it was asked to breathe normally, to relax and to avoid movements as much as possible, so as to minimize artifacts on the acquired data. The Arduino GSR sensor was applied with its power and ground electrodes respectively connected to the index and middle fingers of each subject's left hand, at approximately the height of the last phalanx, as shown in Fig. 3. As a last indication, subjects were asked to place the palm of their hand on the surface of the bed, to improve the coupling and reduce artifacts due to involuntary movements.

Performed acquisitions consisted of two phases: the former, lasting between 10 and 15 min, took place in the absence of audio stimuli to derive the subject's baseline GSR. In the latter phase, each subject listened to 5 audio tracks of different types and duration, played in a randomized order, then expressed how pleasant each listening was, with values from 0 (i.e. no liking at all) to 100 (i.e. extreme satisfaction). The audio tracks used as stimuli belong to the following genres: Track 1 - classical music, Track 2 - jazz music, Track 3 - white noise, Track

4 - rock music, and Track 5 - snoring noise. During both the sessions, subjects were provided with active noise canceling headphones, strongly recommended to improve listening quality and isolate from disturbances.

3.3   Data Processing

According to the Grove-GSR Sensor datasheet [33], the raw GSR data consist of time instants and the corresponding sensor values. Such data were firstly converted into human resistance (i.e. GSR) values, expressed in Ω, according to Eq. (1):

$$GSR[\Omega] = ((1024 + 2 \times SPR) \times 100000)/(512 - SPR), \qquad (1)$$

where SPR stands for Serial Port Reading, i.e., the value displayed on the Serial Port (between 0 and 1023). From the skin resistance values output by the sensor, a conversion to skin conductance (given in µS) may be performed according to Eq. (2):

$$SC[\mu S] = 10^6 * (1/GSR[\Omega]) \qquad (2)$$

Since the GSR signal (and the SC one as well) is an aggregate of two different components, the signals acquired were decomposed into tonic and phasic components. Inspired by the approach described in [23], the tonic component was obtained by applying the basic median filter to the entire signal. In particular, considering sample by sample, the median GSR was computed for each sample and the surrounding samples in the 4 s time interval centred on the current sample (i.e., 80 samples before and after the current one). The phasic component is obtained by subtracting the tonic one from the original GSR signal. Among the most common methods to analyse the phasic component, a classic one is the through-to-peak detection [10,15], which is achieved by finding the onset and

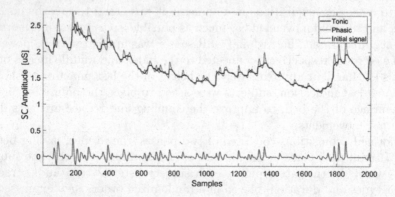

Fig. 4. A sample SC signal generated by processing the Arduino GSR sensor data, and its tonic and phasic components.

offset of signal's peaks. According to the physiological definition of the parameters of phasic electrodermal activity curve [4,23], the onset is generally set to the time point where the curve exceeds a minimum amplitude criterion. Hence, setting two thresholds (peak onset and offset, TH_{ON} and TH_{OFF}) an onset is identified when the signal goes over TH_{ON} and an offset when the signal gets below TH_{OFF}. Then, back to the unfiltered GSR data, the maximum GSR value within each pair of onset and offset is computed and labelled as a GSR peak. From these values, the GSR amplitude is obtained as the difference in signal magnitude at the onset and the peak value.

An example of an SC signal (derived from the GSR one, based on Eq. (2)), from which the phasic and tonic components have been extracted, is shown in Fig. 4.

To analyse the collected data under acoustic stimulation, following the conversion of the values displayed on the Serial Port by the Arduino GSR sensor into GSR (i.e., human resistance), according to Eq. (1), then the initial and the final 10 samples of each acquired signal were removed, to eliminate the transient error and select the GSR data of interest.

4   Results and Discussion

Since everyone has a specific physiological responsiveness at rest, the measured GSR is subjective, depending on the individual. Generally, an initial baseline measurement is carried out for a few minutes, followed by the GSR activity's recording. This procedure allows to identify the so-called *baseline*, that includes individual GSR features and the differences among physiological condition at rest. Moreover, it allows to avoid some issues related to dry skin or undesired environmental stimuli [18]. An example of different neutral baseline signals from two subjects is reported in Fig. 5.

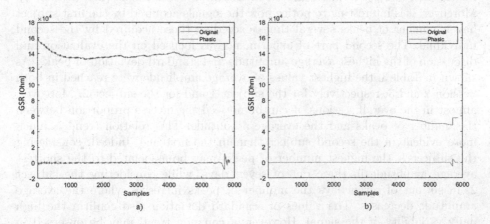

Fig. 5. Baseline of GSR data recorded for a) subject 1, and b) subject 2, during session 4.

Table 1. Number of peaks related to the GSR signals of subject 1.

	Day 1	Day 2	Day 3	Day 4	Day 5	Day 6	Day 7
Session 1	248	**334**	156	**1538**	396	429	389
Session 2	**259**	283	**449**	432	**402**	**464**	381
Session 3	128	251	401	320	356	438	**396**

Table 2. Number of peaks related to the GSR signals of subject 2.

	Day 1	Day 2	Day 3	Day 4	Day 5	Day 6	Day 7
Session 1	219	130	173	185	245	263	139
Session 2	326	**443**	266	237	358	**361**	322
Session 3	**480**	231	**428**	**390**	**394**	315	**389**

Tables 1 and 2 detail the results obtained in the first analysis of this experiment, respectively for the subject 1 and 2. More specifically, in this phase, the number of GSR peaks was counted for each recorded session (i.e., three times per day), and the highest number of peaks achieved in a day was highlighted.

The second analysis was focused on the computation of two statistical figures, namely the average peaks amplitude [μ_p, in Ω] and the corresponding standard deviation [s_p, in Ω]. The weekly results related to the three sessions performed by the two subjects are summarized in Table 3.

In this study, we used the number of peaks on the phasic component as representing the signal physiological content, whereas the mean amplitude of peaks and the corresponding standard deviation metrics were considered for a quantitative analysis of the GSR signal variations.

As underlined in Tables 1 and 2, while the highest number of peaks for the second subject was mainly achieved in the evening sessions (i.e., Session 2), for the first subject it was achieved in the afternoon sessions (i.e., Session 3). Moreover, it is interesting to notice how the signals acquired by the first subject had a number of peaks several times exceeding those acquired by the second individual. The second part of experiment was focused on the evaluation and discussion of the highest average amplitude and standard deviation of peaks. As shown in Table 3, the highest values of average amplitude were reached in both Session 2 and 3, respectively for the subject 1 and for the subject 2. Moreover, almost in the overall sessions, it can be noticed the inverse proportion between the number of peaks and the average amplitude. This relation trend is much more evident in the second subject than in the first one. Indeed, considering the subject 1, the highest number of peaks may be associated to the shortest average amplitude in three out of seven days, while considering the subject 2, in six out of seven days the number of peaks increases where the average amplitude decreases. The values of standard deviation also confirm the high daily variability of the signal. However, a common trend may be observed in the majority of days. In fact, almost in the overall session, both the subjects showed the highest standard deviation in the morning acquisition. Contrarily,

Table 3. Average Amplitude (μ_p, in Ω) and Standard Deviation (s_p, in Ω) of GSR peak values, related to both subject 1 (on the left) and subject 2 (on the right).

Day	Session	μ_p [Ω]	s_p [Ω]	Day	Session	μ_p [Ω]	s_p [Ω]
	Session 1	85.7	296.3		Session 1	87.4	260.4
Day 1	Session 2	40.4	441.5	Day 1	Session 2	11.1	98.3
	Session 3	174.2	330.7		Session 3	4.8	41.4
	Session 1	71.8	366.9		Session 1	184.5	376.7
Day 2	Session 2	17.2	79.8	Day 2	Session 2	8.1	130.3
	Session 3	31.9	116.4		Session 3	17.7	63.8
	Session 1	483.2	1.1×10^3		Session 1	139.8	293.3
Day 3	Session 2	22.3	168.2	Day 3	Session 2	19.2	83.3
	Session 3	18.7	163.4		Session 3	4.3	53.3
	Session 1	64.1	493.9		Session 1	56.7	152.7
Day 4	Session 2	7.0	144.8	Day 4	Session 2	141.6	370.8
	Session 3	27.9	198.5		Session 3	1.6	22.2
	Session 1	14.6	234.1		Session 1	46.5	134.4
Day 5	Session 2	30.5	205.8	Day 5	Session 2	19.4	114.4
	Session 3	212.4	2.9×10^3		Session 3	3.6	37.3
	Session 1	34.3	318.8		Session 1	100.6	354.2
Day 6	Session 2	42.5	417.2	Day 6	Session 2	11.7	65.5
	Session 3	0	0		Session 3	19.5	77.9
	Session 1	23.3	460.3		Session 1	104.3	214.3
Day 7	Session 2	22.1	162.6	Day 7	Session 2	13.6	89.8
	Session 3	19.4	157.6		Session 3	28.7	321.3

Table 4. Mean value (μ) and standard deviation (s) of the GSR, and percent pleasure value (Ple.), for each track and subject.

	Subject 1			Subject 2			Subject 3			Subject 4			Subject 5			Subject 6		
	GSR μ [Ω]	GSR s [Ω]	Ple. [%]	GSR μ [Ω]	GSR s [Ω]	Ple. [%]	GSR μ [Ω]	GSR s [Ω]	Ple. [%]	GSR μ [Ω]	GSR s [Ω]	Ple. [%]	GSR μ [Ω]	GSR s [Ω]	Ple. [%]	GSR μ [Ω]	GSR s [Ω]	Ple [%]
Baseline	493	8	--	437	15	-	336	16	-	140	36	-	426	4	-	445	3	-
Track 1	474	13	85	385	41	55	342	22	10	249	48	55	438	3	100	428	1	100
Track 2	466	14	100	429	24	30	350	17	80	235	51	65	424	15	100	391	11	90
Track 3	466	10	40	318	29	10	313	13	0	225	18	4	330	20	5	365	20	10
Track 4	471	10	60	407	20	70	315	13	80	198	68	60	380	28	70	415	14	80
Track 5	461	8	30	334	29	0	294	15	0	172	17	0	338	18	0	364	26	0

analysing the remaining standard deviation values, the subject 1 achieved the lowest values mainly in the session 2 while the subject 2 in the session 3. The outcomes confirm as the GSR is a daily changing signal, reflecting the variability in electrical resistance of the skin related to sweating.

For the analysis of the skin resistance variations due to acoustic stimulation, the mean and standard deviation values of the GSR were computed, for each acquired GSR data series corresponding to each subject, both in the baseline condition and during each audio track listening. Additionally, for each subject, the difference in absolute value between the mean GSR measured in the baseline, and

Table 5. Difference between the mean GSR value corresponding to the track listening (μ_t) and the mean GSR value of the baseline (μ_b), and percent pleasure value (Ple.) for the track, for all the subjects. The bold numbers correspond to the two highest mean GSR difference values, for each subject.

Track	Subject 1		Subject 2		Subject 3		Subject 4		Subject 5		Subject 6	
	$\mu_t - \mu_b$ [Ω]	Ple. [%]	$\mu_t - \mu_b$ [Ω]	Ple. [%]	$\mu_t - \mu_b$ [Ω]	Ple. [%]	$\mu_t - \mu_b$ [Ω]	Ple. [%]	$\mu_t - \mu_b$ [Ω]	Ple. [%]	$\mu_t - \mu_b$ [Ω]	Ple. [%]
Track 1	19	85	52	55	5	10	**109**	55	13	100	17	100
Track 2	**27**	100	7	30	14	80	**95**	65	2	100	54	90
Track 3	**27**	40	**119**	10	**23**	0	85	4	**96**	5	**79**	10
Track 4	22	60	29	70	21	80	58	60	46	70	30	80
Track 5	**32**	30	**103**	0	**43**	0	32	0	**87**	0	**81**	0

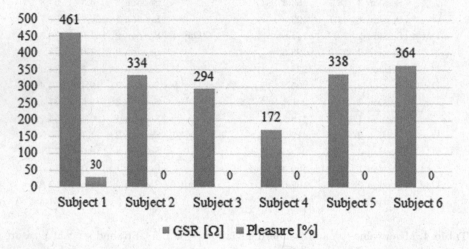

Fig. 6. Mean values of GSR, and percent pleasure during Track 5 reproduction, for the 6 subjects.

the mean GSR measured during acoustic stimulation, was computed, with the aim of evaluating the variations of the signal with respect to the reference condition.

Table 4 shows the experimental results in terms of mean value (μ) and standard deviation (s) of the GSR for every track and every subject, compared to the values measured for each subject in the baseline. Table 5 shows the difference between the mean GSR during each track stimulation, and the mean GSR measured for the baseline. In both the tables, also the pleasure felt during the listening experience, and expressed in percent values, is provided, for each subject and audio track. As it can be seen in the tables, Track 3 and Track 5, that are white noise and snoring noise respectively, present the lowest scores pleasure. This result is reflected also in the difference values of Table 5. In fact, for Track 3 and Track 5 the difference is higher for every subject, except for subject 4. Moreover, Fig. 6 shows the mean values of the GSR and the pleasure scores for every subject reported in Table 4, but only for Track 5 (i.e., snoring noise), that is the track with the lowest pleasure scores, and for which a highest difference between mean GSR values is found in 5 subjects out of 6.

These results, despite not being generalizable because of the limited number of tests participants, show that the impact of the audio stimuli on a subject is more evident when unpleasant sounds (white noise and snoring noise, in the cases under study) are involved. On the contrary, there is no evident correlation between GSR values and pleasant tracks (with pleasure > 80). In fact, for some subjects a pleasure of 100% corresponds to a high difference on mean GSR (e.g., subject 1), while for other subjects it is related to a low difference on mean GSR (e.g., subject 5 and subject 6).

5   Conclusion

In order to investigate the individual GSR features, it is crucial to compare the individual baseline of GSR activity and the stimuli-evoked reactions. However, many studies omit the research of GSR in physical and mental rest conditions. For this reason, this work proposes an experimental approach that allows to explore the GSR data recorded at rest condition, by means of a portable low-cost and easy-to-use device.

Firstly, the analysis went through a qualitative approach, finding the relationship between the number of peaks and the trends of GSR signal recorded by two different subjects at rest. Since the GSR is a subjective signal and measurement, it is very difficult to perform a comparison between different subjects, especially due to their own skin resistance with individual basis threshold and peaks [14]. The findings of this study, despite not being generalizable because of the limited number of test participants, suggest that the impact of the acoustic stimuli on a subject is more evident when unpleasant sounds are involved. Additional research should be performed to clarify the effects associated to sounds perceived as pleasant.

The outcomes of our exploration can be considered promising for future analysis. Some developments might regard the extraction of GSR features to classify emotional response in reaction to external audio stimuli and compared to a self-assessment questionnaire. Moreover, future works should focus on expanding the validation and the reliability of the investigated experimental approach, involving a larger population.

References

1. Amidei, A., et al.: Driver drowsiness detection based on variation of skin conductance from wearable device. In: 2022 IEEE International Workshop on Metrology for Automotive (MetroAutomotive), pp. 94–98 (2022). https://doi.org/10.1109/MetroAutomotive54295.2022.9854871
2. Appler, J.M., Goodrich, L.V.: Connecting the ear to the brain: molecular mechanisms of auditory circuit assembly. Prog. Neurobiol. **93**(4), 488–508 (2011)

3. Baracskai, Z., Finn, S.: Relaxation effects of binaural phenomena. In: Audio Engineering Society Conference: 52nd International Conference: Sound Field Control-Engineering and Perception. Audio Engineering Society (2013)
4. Boucsein, W.: Parameters of Phasic Electrodermal Activity, pp. 151–158. Springer (2012)
5. Can, Y., Chalabianloo, N., Ekiz, D., Ersoy, C.: Continuous stress detection using wearable sensors in real life: Algorithmic programming contest case study. Sensors **19**, 1849 (2019)
6. Chanda, M.L., Levitin, D.J.: The neurochemistry of music. Trends Cogn. Sci. **17**(4), 179–193 (2013)
7. Chatterjee, D., Gavas, R., Saha, S.K.: Exploring skin conductance features for cross-subject emotion recognition. In: 2022 IEEE Region 10 Symposium (TENSYMP), pp. 1–6 (2022). https://doi.org/10.1109/TENSYMP54529.2022.9864492
8. Christidis, D., Kalliris, G., Papanikolaou, G., Sevastiadis, C., Dimoulas, C.: Development of an engineering application for subjective evaluation of human response to noise. In: Audio Engineering Society Convention 110. Audio Engineering Society (2001)
9. Christoforou, C., Christou-Champi, S., Constantinidou, F., Theodorou, M.: From the eyes and the heart: a novel eye-gaze metric that predicts video preferences of a large audience. Front. Psychol. **6**, 579 (2015)
10. Cowley, B.U., Torniainen, J.: A short review and primer on electrodermal activity in human computer interaction applications. CoRR **1608** (06986v3) (2016)
11. Daponte, P., De Vito, L., Iadarola, G., Picariello, F.: ECG monitoring based on dynamic compressed sensing of multi-lead signals. Sensors **21**(21), 7003 (2021). https://doi.org/10.3390/s21217003
12. Dourou, N., Bruschi, V., Spinsante, S., Cecchi, S.: The influence of listeners' mood on equalization-based listening experience. Acoustics **4**(3), 746–763 (2022). https://doi.org/10.3390/acoustics4030045
13. Dourou, N., Poli, A., Terenzi, A., Cecchi, S., Spinsante, S.: IoT-enabled analysis of subjective sound quality perception based on out-of-lab physiological measurements. In: Spinsante, S., Silva, B., Goleva, R. (eds.) HealthyIoT 2021. LNICST, vol. 432, pp. 153–165. Springer, Cham (2022). https://doi.org/10.1007/978-3-030-99197-5_13
14. Foglia, P., Prete, C.A., Zanda, M.: Relating GSR signals to traditional usability metrics: case study with an anthropomorphic web assistant. In: 2008 IEEE Instrumentation and Measurement Technology Conference, pp. 1814–1818 (2008)
15. Gautam, A., Simoes-Capela, N., Schiavone, G., Acharyya, A., De Raedt, W., Van Hoof, C.: A data driven empirical iterative algorithm for GSR signal pre-processing. In: 2018 26th European Signal Processing Conference (EUSIPCO) (2018). https://doi.org/10.23919/EUSIPCO.2018.8553191
16. Greco, A., Valenza, G., Citi, L., Scilingo, E.P.: Arousal and valence recognition of affective sounds based on electrodermal activity. IEEE Sens. J. **17**(3), 716–725 (2016)
17. Healey, J.A., Picard, R.W.: Detecting stress during real-world driving tasks using physiological sensors. IEEE Trans. Intell. Transp. Syst. **6**(2), 156–166 (2005). https://doi.org/10.1109/TITS.2005.848368
18. Hogan, J.N., Baucom, B.R.: Behavioral, affective, and physiological monitoring, pp. 7–10. Academic Press (2016)
19. Hudspeth, A.J.: How the ear's works work. Nature **341**(6241), 397–404 (1989)

20. Iadarola, G., Poli, A., Spinsante, S.: Analysis of galvanic skin response to acoustic stimuli by wearable devices. In: 2021 IEEE International Symposium on Medical Measurements and Applications (MeMeA), pp. 1–6. IEEE (2021)

21. Iadarola, G., Poli, A., Spinsante, S.: Reconstruction of galvanic skin response peaks via sparse representation. In: 2021 IEEE International Instrumentation and Measurement Technology Conference (I2MTC), pp. 1–6 (2021). https://doi.org/10.1109/I2MTC50364.2021.9459905

22. Iadarola, G., Poli, A., Spinsante, S.: Compressed sensing of skin conductance level for IoT-based wearable sensors. In: 2022 IEEE International Instrumentation and Measurement Technology Conference (I2MTC), pp. 1–6 (2022). https://doi.org/10.1109/I2MTC48687.2022.9806516

23. iMotions: Galvanic skin response (GSR): the complete pocket guide (2016). https://imotions.com/blog/galvanic-skin-response/

24. Jambhale, K., et al.: Selection of optimal physiological features for accurate detection of stress. In: 2022 44th Annual International Conference of the IEEE Engineering in Medicine & Biology Society (EMBC), pp. 2514–2517 (2022). https://doi.org/10.1109/EMBC48229.2022.9871067

25. Juslin, P.N., Sloboda, J.: Handbook of music and emotion: theory, research, applications. Oxford University Press, New York (2011)

26. Juslin, P.N., Västfjäll, D.: Emotional responses to music: the need to consider underlying mechanisms. Behav. Brain Sci. **31**(5), 559–575 (2008)

27. Kyriakou, K., et al.: Detecting moments of stress from measurements of wearable physiological sensors. Sensors **19**(17), 3805 (2019). https://doi.org/10.3390/s19173805

28. Poli, A., Brocanelli, A., Cecchi, S., Orcioni, S., Spinsante, S.: Preliminary results of IoT-enabled EDA-based analysis of physiological response to acoustic stimuli. In: Goleva, R., Garcia, N.R.C., Pires, I.M. (eds.) HealthyIoT 2020. LNICST, vol. 360, pp. 124–136. Springer, Cham (2021). https://doi.org/10.1007/978-3-030-69963-5_9

29. Poli, A., Cecchi, S., Spinsante, S., Terenzi, A., Bettarelli, F.: A preliminary study on the correlation between subjective sound quality perception and physiological parameters. In: Audio Engineering Society Convention 150. Audio Engineering Society (2021)

30. Qin, Y., Zhang, H., Wang, Y., Mao, M., Chen, F.: 3D music impact on autonomic nervous system response and its therapeutic potential. In: 2020 IEEE Conference On Multimedia Information Processing and Retrieval (MIPR), pp. 364–369. IEEE (2020)

31. Rentfrow, P.J., Goldberg, L.R., Levitin, D.J.: The structure of musical preferences: a five-factor model. J. Pers. Soc. Psychol. **100**(6), 1139 (2011)

32. Schilk, P., Dheman, K., Magno, M.: VitalPod: a low power in-ear vital parameter monitoring system. In: 2022 18th International Conference on Wireless and Mobile Computing, Networking and Communications (WiMob), pp. 94–99 (2022). https://doi.org/10.1109/WiMob55322.2022.9941646

33. Seeed: Grove-GSR sensor (2010). https://wiki.seeedstudio.com/Grove-GSR_Sensor/

34. Sharma, V., Prakash, N.R., Kalra, P.: Audio-video emotional response mapping based upon electrodermal activity. Biomed. Signal Process. Control **47**, 324–333 (2019)

35. Shen, W., et al.: Subjective evaluation of personalized equalization curves in music. In: Audio Engineering Society Convention 133. Audio Engineering Society (2012)

36. Sudheesh, N., Joseph, K.: Investigation into the effects of music and meditation on galvanic skin response. ITBM-RBM **21**(3), 158–163 (2000)

37. Weninger, F., Eyben, F., Schuller, B.W., Mortillaro, M., Scherer, K.R.: On the acoustics of emotion in audio: what speech, music, and sound have in common. Front. Psychol. **4**, 292 (2013)

38. Williams, D., Wu, C.Y., Hodge, V., Murphy, D., Cowling, P.: A psychometric evaluation of emotional responses to horror music. In: Audio Engineering Society Convention 146. Audio Engineering Society (2019)

39. Yang, W., et al.: Affective auditory stimulus database: An expanded version of the international affective digitized sounds (iads-e). Behav. Res. Methods **50**(4), 1415–1429 (2018)

40. Zhang, K., Zhang, H., Li, S., Yang, C., Sun, L.: The PMEmo dataset for music emotion recognition. In: Proceedings of the 2018 ACM on International Conference on Multimedia Retrieval, pp. 135–142 (2018)

41. Zhang, T., El Ali, A., Wang, C., Hanjalic, A., Cesar, P.: CorrNet: fine-grained emotion recognition for video watching using wearable physiological sensors. Sensors **21**(1), 52 (2021). https://doi.org/10.3390/s21010052,https://www.mdpi.com/1424-8220/21/1/52

IoT Applications in Research and Clinical Practice

Multivariate Classification of Mild and Moderate Hearing Loss Using a Speech-in-Noise Test for Hearing Screening at a Distance

Edoardo Maria Polo[1] , Maximiliano Mollura[2] , Riccardo Barbieri[2] ,
and Alessia Paglialonga[3]([✉])

[1] DIAG, Università la Sapienza di Roma, 00185 Rome, Italy
[2] Dipartimento di Elettronica, Informazione e Bioingegneria (DEIB), Politecnico di Milano, 20133 Milan, Italy
[3] Cnr-Istituto di Elettronica e di Ingegneria dell'Informazione e delle Telecomunicazioni (CNR-IEIIT), 20133 Milan, Italy
alessia.paglialonga@ieiit.cnr.it

Abstract. In the area of smartphone-based hearing screening, the number of speech-in-noise tests available is growing rapidly. However, the available tests are typically based on a univariate classification approach, for example using the speech recognition threshold (SRT) or the number of correct responses. There is still lack of multivariate approaches to screen for hearing loss (HL). Moreover, all the screening methods developed so far do not assess the degree of HL, despite the potential importance of this information in terms of patient education and clinical follow-up. The aim of this study was to characterize multivariate approaches to identify mild and moderate HL using a recently developed, validated speech-in-noise test for hearing screening at a distance, namely the WHISPER (Widespread Hearing Impairment Screening and PrEvention of Risk) test. The WHISPER test is automated, minimally dependent on the listeners' native language, it is based on an optimized, efficient adaptive procedure, and it uses a multivariate approach. The results showed that age and SRT were the features with highest performance in identifying mild and moderate HL, respectively. Multivariate classifiers using all the WHISPER features achieved better performance than univariate classifiers, reaching an accuracy equal to 0.82 and 0.87 for mild and moderate HL, respectively. Overall, this study suggested that mild and moderate HL may be discriminated with high accuracy using a set of features extracted from the WHISPER test, laying the ground for the development of future self-administered speech-in-noise tests able to provide specific recommendations based on the degree of HL.

Keywords: Hearing loss · Hearing screening · Machine learning · Smartphone-based screening · Multivariate classifiers

S. Spinsante et al. (Eds.): HealthyIoT 2022, LNICST 456, pp. 81–92, 2023.
https://doi.org/10.1007/978-3-031-28663-6_7

1 Introduction

In the growing field of mobile health (mHealth), a number of smartphone hearing health apps have been developed for a variety of purposes, e.g., hearing screening, hearing aid management, patient education, and hearing rehabilitation [1–5]. Hearing screening is becoming increasingly popular as a means to increase awareness and identify the earlier signs of age-related hearing loss (HL), which would be typically left unnoticed otherwise [6, 7]. Among the validated apps introduced for adult hearing screening, some use pure-tone audiometry whereas others use speech-in-noise testing. The interest around speech-in-noise screening tests is growing as they can help detect real-life communication problems, for example difficulties in having conversations in noisy environments. Moreover, differently than pure tone audiometry, speech-in-noise tests are less sensitive to calibration procedures and can be performed in uncontrolled noise environments [8–11].

Recently, we have developed and validated a novel, automated speech-in-noise screening test viable for testing at a distance, e.g., through a web- or mobile-app, namely the WHISPER test (Widespread Hearing Impairment Screening and PrEvention of Risk) [12–16]. Differently than the majority of currently available speech-in-noise tests, the WHISPER test is minimally dependent on the listeners' native language, it is based on an optimized, efficient adaptive procedure, and it extracts a list of variables in addition to the speech recognition threshold (SRT), that is the most common variable used for speech-based screening [12–15, 17]. Multivariate approaches to HL identification such as the one used in the WHISPER test may help overcome the limitations of univariate approaches based on SRT only. In fact, individuals with normal hearing may have poor SRTs, whereas individuals with HL may be able to reach satisfactory speech recognition performance [18, 19]. Moreover, research has shown that features such as the subject's age or the average reaction time can help identify HL [13, 17, 18, 20, 21]. Nevertheless, multivariate approaches to HL identification and classification are not widely adopted yet.

In our previous studies, we have assessed the ability of multivariate approaches to identify HL of mild degree or higher, using both the former and the newer World Health Organization (WHO) definitions of HL (i.e., average value of pure-tone thresholds at 0.5, 1, 2, and 4 kHz (PTA) higher than 25 dB HL and higher than 20 dB HL, respectively [22, 23]). Specifically, in a preliminary sample of 148 participants (age $= 52.1 \pm 20.4$ years; age range: 20–89 years; 46 males, 102 female), we showed that multivariate classifiers based on, for example, logistic regression (LR), support vector machines, k-nearest neighbors, or random forest were more accurate than univariate classifiers to identify HL of mild degree or higher, using the former WHO definition of HL [13, 15]. In the same sample of participants, we showed that LR was also able to accurately predict the self-perceived hearing handicap, as measured using the Hearing Handicap Inventory for the Elderly–Screening Version (HHIE-S) [17]. In a larger sample of 207 participants (age $= 52 \pm 20$ years; age range: 20–89 years; 66 males, 141 female), we confirmed that multivariate classifiers could achieve high accuracy (up to 0.85 with RF) and we showed, using post-hoc explainability techniques, that he most important features for the identification of mild HL, using the newer WHO definition, were age, SRT, average reaction time, and percentage of correct responses [17].

In all the above studies, multivariate algorithms were characterized considering binary classification of two output classes, i.e., normal hearing vs HL (mild or higher). Whereas binary classification can be appropriate for general HL detection, nevertheless knowledge of the degree of HL (e.g., mild-to-moderate vs moderate) would be important, particularly for hearing screening delivered at a distance using unsupervised tests via web or smartphone. In fact, individuals with different degrees of HL should undergo different intervention strategies and should be provided with different follow-up information and educational content [24]. The aim of this study was to characterize, for the first time, multivariate approaches to identify mild and moderate HL (mild HL: 20 dB HL < PTA ≤ 40 dB HL; moderate HL: PTA > 40 dB HL) using the WHISPER test.

The article is organized as follows. Section 2 outlines the study participants and protocol and the data analysis approach used. Section 3 presents the results obtained in terms of univariate and multivariate feature characterization and classification performances for binary and multi-class classification (NH vs mild-to-moderate HL vs moderate HL). Section 4 discusses the obtained results in the context of the available literature. Finally, the conclusions of the study and the possible future developments are outlined in Sect. 5.

2 Methods

2.1 Participants and Procedure

The study sample included 350 participants (117 men, 223 women; age: mean 49 years, range: 18–89 years) tested during HL awareness events. The study dataset includes 442 records (92 participants tested in both ears, 258 in one ear).

Pure-tone audiometry was performed at 0.5, 1, 2, and 4 kHz (Amplaid 177+ by Amplifon, TDH49 headphones) and speech-in-noise testing using the WHISPER test. Testing was performed in a quiet room at hearing screening and awareness initiatives. The protocol was approved by the Politecnico di Milano Research Ethical Committee (Opinion No. 2/2019, Feb 19, 2019; renewed by Opinion No. 13/2022, Apr 13, 2022).

The WHISPER test is delivered on a touch-screen interface and is based on an adaptive procedure. Specifically, a sequence of meaningless vowel–consonant–vowel (VCV) syllables (e.g., ata and asa) are presented at varying signal-to-noise ratio (SNR) in a three-alternative multiple-choice paradigm. Further details on the WHISPER test are reported in [12, 15, 21]. The following features were extracted from the WHISPER test: SRT, number of correct responses (#correct), percentage of correct responses (%correct), average reaction time, and test duration.

2.2 Data Analysis

The ears tested were classified in three classes, following the WHO definitions of mild and moderate HL [22, 23]. Specifically, the following three classes were defined: (i) normal hearing (NH): PTA ≤ 20 dB HL; 299 ears (~68%); (ii) mild HL: 20 dB HL < PTA ≤ 40 dB HL; 97 ears (~22%); and (iii) moderate HL: PTA > 40 dB HL; 46 ears (~10%). Six input features were considered for classification, i.e., the five features extracted from the WHISPER test and the subject's age.

Univariate and Multivariate Characterization of Features. The Receiver Operating Characteristics (ROC) for binary classification (i.e., mild HL vs NH; and moderate HL vs NH) were computed for each of the six input features and for LR on two combinations of features, i.e.: (i) the full set of six features and (ii) a subset of features with AUC $\geq$ 0.80 for *both* mild HL vs NH and moderate HL vs NH classification. The LR algorithm was used following results from [15, 17].

The Shapiro-Wilk test was performed to check for normality of the distributions of the six input features in the three output classes. As the distributions were not normal, possible differences in median values between the three classes were assessed using the Kruskal-Wallis test with Bonferroni correction. A significance level $\alpha = 0.05$ was considered.

Binary and Multiclass Classification Performance. Classification performance was assessed by training a LR algorithm for binary classification (mild HL vs NL, moderate HL vs NH) and multi-class classification (NH vs mild HL vs moderate HL). The data set was randomly split into a training set including 80% of the sample (353 records) and a test set including the remaining 20% (89 records). Stratification was applied to maintain the same percentage of records in the two classes of the original data set in the training and test partitions. Class weights were applied to the data to compute LR coefficients to limit the effect of class imbalance, particularly for the moderate HL class. Data were standardized to zero mean and unit variance. Due to the relatively small size of the data set, 5-fold cross-validation was introduced on the training set to partially reduce the influence of the selected partition on the trained model.

3   Results

Figure 1 shows the distributions of the six input features in the three output classes (NH, mild HL, and moderate HL). Age, SRT, and average reaction time tended to increase with increasing degree of HL. All the observed differences in median values of age, SRT, and average reaction time were statistically significant, except for the age difference between mild and moderate HL. The features #correct and %correct tended to decrease with increasing degree of HL. All the observed differences in median values of #correct and %correct were statistically significant. The test duration tended to increase from NH to mild HL, but not from NH or mild HL to moderate HL.

Figure 2 shows the ROC estimated using, for each HL class, the feature with highest performance (age and SRT for mild and moderate HL, respectively) and using LR on (i) the full set of six features and (ii) a subset of features with AUC $\geq$ 0.80, i.e. age, SRT, and average reaction time. The univariate and multivariate performance of each feature and feature combinations for mild HL vs NH classification and for moderate HL vs NH classification is shown in Table 1 and Table 2, respectively.

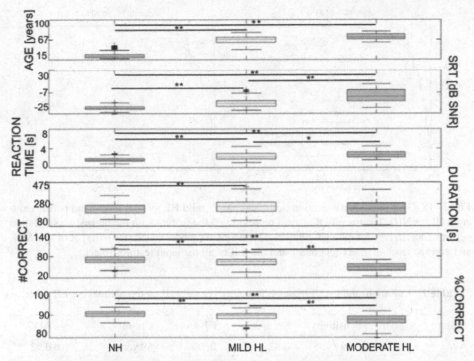

Fig. 1. Distribution of features in the three output classes: normal hearing, mild HL, and moderate HL. Statistically significant differences in median values between the classes are marked with * (p < 0.05) and ** (p < 0.01).

The feature with the highest performance for mild HL identification was age, whereas the one with highest performance for moderate HL identification was SRT (accuracy = 0.86 at the optimal cut-off value). For moderate HL identification, the performance of age was lower than that of SRT but still relatively high (accuracy = 0.82). The optimal cut-off values for age, SRT, average reaction time, and test duration increased from mild to moderate HL, whereas those for %correct and #correct decreased with increasing degree of HL, in line with the trends shown in Fig. 1. Using LR on combinations of three or six features did not lead to improved performance for mild HL identification, as shown in Table 1. For moderate HL identification, LR on three and on six features achieved improved performance (accuracy up to 0.90). In general, the highest performance for *both* mild HL and moderate HL identification was observed using LR on the full set of six features.

Table 3 shows the observed performance of LR for binary and multiclass classification performance, as measured in the training set (average ± s.d. from 5-fold cross validation) and in the test set. The observed accuracies were higher than 0.81 for binary classification and equal to 0.72 for multiclass classification, with no remarkable differences in performance between the average performance on the training set and the estimated performance on the test set, suggesting no overfitting effects. For binary classification, both sensitivity and specificity were high, indicating very good performance.

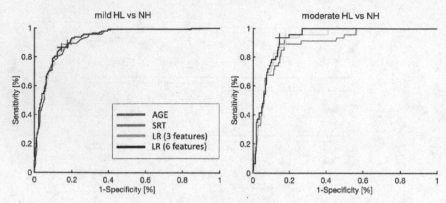

Fig. 2. ROC for binary classification (left-hand panel: mild HL vs NH; right-hand panel: moderate HL vs NH). The three ROC shown represent: (i) the feature with the highest classification performance, i.e. age for mild HL (dark blue) and SRT for moderate HL (red); (ii) LR of age, SRT, and average reaction time (light blue); and (iii) LR of all the input features (black).

Table 1. Univariate and multivariate performance for mild HL at the optimal cut-off value.

Feature	Sensitivity	Specificity	F1-score	Cut-off	AUC
Age	0.89	0.83	0.78	59 years	0.92
SRT	0.78	0.76	0.68	−12.14 dB SNR	0.85
Avg reaction time	0.74	0.75	0.64	1.9 s	0.80
Duration	0.57	0.61	0.48	252 s	0.58
%Correct	0.64	0.70	0.43	0.90	0.75
#Correct	0.67	0.66	0.44	66	0.74
LR (3 features)	0.86	0.86	0.79	–	0.92
LR (6 features)	0.87	0.86	0.80	–	0.93

The sensitivity in multiclass classification was lower compared to binary classification, in line with the higher number of classes. Nevertheless, multiclass classification performance was still good as sensitivity was around 0.70 and specificity was around 0.85. The lower values of sensitivity, specificity, and accuracy measured in the test set shown in Table 3 compared to those measured at the optimal cut-off value using the ROC (Table 1, Table 2) are related to the use of machine learning, as opposed to simple ROC analysis, and to the relatively small size of the dataset that leads to the observed variability in performance due to the underlying uncertainty in data. This variability is demonstrated by the observed standard deviation of the accuracy on the training set across 5-fold cross validation (s.d. up to ± 0.05). The higher values of F1-score observed for moderate HL vs NH classification compared to those shown in Table 2 may be related to the use of class weights that may have partially compensated the effect of class imbalance on F1-score estimates.

Table 2. Univariate and multivariate performance for moderate HL at the optimal cut-off value.

Feature	Sensitivity	Specificity	F1-score	Cut-off	AUC
Age	0.83	0.81	0.48	67 years	0.89
SRT	0.89	0.82	0.52	−7.48 dB SNR	0.89
Avg reaction time	0.83	0.72	0.38	2.20 s	0.83
Duration	0.41	0.70	0.19	274 s	0.49
%Correct	0.80	0.74	0.23	0.89	0.80
#Correct	0.82	0.78	0.24	60	0.88
LR (3 features)	0.93	0.82	0.52	–	0.92
LR (6 features)	0.93	0.86	0.57	–	0.93

Table 3. Binary and multiclass classification performance using LR.

	Accuracy (training)	Accuracy (test)	F1-score (training)	F1-score (test)	Sens (test)	Spec (test)
Mild HL/NH	0.84 ± 0.05	0.81	0.83 ± 0.06	0.79	0.83	0.80
Moderate HL/NH	0.85 ± 0.02	0.84	0.72 ± 0.03	0.72	0.89	0.84
Moderate HL/mild HL/NH	0.74 ± 0.04	0.72	0.63 ± 0.05	0.64	0.69	0.85

4 Discussion

The availability of methods for accurate identification of the degree of HL (i.e., mild vs moderate) following hearing screening via unsupervised tests delivered through web- or mobile- platforms would be important for tailoring clinical assessment and patient education. Nevertheless, current univariate approaches typically target mild HL. Also, there is still lack of multivariate approaches able to discriminate the degree of HL using a speech-in-noise screening test. In this study, we characterized the univariate and multivariate performance of a set of six features extracted from the WHISPER speech-in-noise screening test for the sake of identifying mild and moderate HL in unscreened adults.

Results in Fig. 1, Table 1, and Table 2 indicated that the univariate classification performance of the six features extracted from the WHISPER platform varied with varying degree of hearing loss. Specifically, the features with higher performance (i.e., AUC ≥ 0.80) for mild HL identification were age, SRT, and average reaction time. The features with higher performance for moderate HL identification were age, SRT, #Correct, average reaction time, and %correct. The highest accuracy at the optimal ROC point was observed using age and a cut-off value equal to 59 years for mild HL and using SRT and a cut-off value equal to -7.48 dB SNR for moderate HL. Age and SRT were the features with higher performance for both mild and moderate HL (AUC $\geq$ 0.85), followed by average reaction time (AUC $\geq$ 0.80). The cut-off value for age, SRT, and average reaction time increased with increasing degree of HL. The feature with the lowest classification performance was test duration (AUC $= 0.58$ and 0.49 for mild and moderate HL, respectively).

The relationship between SRT, pure-tone thresholds, and age is well known. Age-related deficits in auditory and cognitive processing may play a role when speech is presented in background noise such as in the proposed screening test [18, 25, 26]. As shown in our earlier study, the interaction between age and PTA can accurately predict SRT [12], in line with the fact that the ability to properly recognize speech is the result of complex relationships between age, degree of HL, and cognitive abilities [27, 28]. The relevance of the average reaction time was also highlighted in previous studies in relation to mild HL detection [13, 17] and it is confirmed here for both mild and moderate HL classification. Regarding test duration, the univariate classification abilities were, in general, poor, with negligible differences in the distributions of test duration across the three classes. This may be interpreted in light of a compensation effect related to the adaptive nature of the WHISPER procedure. In fact, individuals with increasing degree of HL have in general poorer speech recognition abilities and worse cognitive abilities and, as such, they tend to exhibit longer reaction times when responding to a given stimulus in the trial. However, individuals with poorer speech recognition performance tend to go through a lower number of trials in the adaptive procedure as the staircase reaches convergence earlier if there is a high number of incorrect responses [12, 15, 17].

Multivariate characterization of features indicated that the classification performance obtained using LR on age, SRT, and average reaction time (i.e., the three features with AUC $\geq$ 0.80 for both mild and moderate HL) and the one obtained using LR on the full set of six features led to increased performance compared to the best univariate feature. LR on the six features yielded the highest performance for both mild and moderate HL classification. These results suggest that a multivariate approach may be more accurate than the best-performing univariate ones in discriminating different degrees of HL from the speech-in-noise test here used. The accuracy obtained by training a ML classifier using the six features was 0.82 and 0.87 for mild and moderate HL, respectively, suggesting high classification performance (Table 3).

The observed multivariate classification performance was equal to or higher than that observed in previous studies or with other speech-in-noise tests. For example, identification of mild HL using the SRT estimated from English digits-in-noise test yielded an accuracy equal to 0.82 [29]. In our previous study, using data from a smaller sample of 207 participants, we observed an accuracy equal to 0.86 for mild HL using the full set of six features [17]. The slightly lower accuracy observed in the current study may be related to differences in the underlying data and classification approach. Specifically, in [17] records with mild and moderate HL were aggregated in a single HL class, the output classes NH and HL were balanced (54% vs 46%), and age was more strongly correlated with HL. In a recent study, multiclass classification performance of the digits-in-noise test was assessed using a univariate approach based on the estimated SRT in a large sample of 3422 participants from the Rotterdam study. The observed accuracy at the optimal ROC point was 0.72 for mild HL (42% of the sample) and 0.95 for moderate HL (12% of the sample) [30]. Another study assessed self-conducted SRT measured using the German matrix sentence test in home settings against two criteria for HL, i.e. (i) the earlier WHO criterion for mild HL (i.e., PTA > 25 dB HL), and (ii) the German criterion for hearing aid indication (i.e., pure-tone threshold > 30 dB in one or more frequencies between 500 Hz and 4 kHz), that is similar to a moderate HL criterion [31]. The study showed that the accuracy for criterion (i) was 0.74 whereas that of criterion (ii) was 0.76, i.e., lower than the performance here observed with our multivariate approach.

The study here shown has some limitations. First, the distribution of age and degree of HL in our sample may not reflect that of the general population. For example, in our sample we observed a prevalence of HL equal to 32% that is higher than the reported prevalence of hearing loss in adults, i.e., about 20% [32]. This sampling bias may be related to the experiment settings whereby data were collected primarily within the context of hearing screening and awareness initiatives for the general public. For similar reasons, the sample may have been biased towards higher age than that of the general population. It will be important in future studies to limit the sampling bias and assess the univariate and multivariate classification performance in a larger sample including a higher proportion of individuals with NH and a higher proportion of middle aged and young adults. In addition, our multivariate approach was based on a set of only six features extracted from the WHISPER test. It will be interesting to investigate further features, for example those related to psychometric functions estimated from the adaptive procedure, or individual performance in subsets of stimuli (e.g., high-frequency vs low-frequency stimuli), or more complex measures of reaction time. Inclusion of a cognitive testing module into the WHISPER platform could also help address in more detail the relationships between hearing sensitivity, speech recognition, reaction time, and aging. Last, but not least, in this study we focused on the WHISPER test only. It will be important to investigate univariate and multivariate classification performance towards mild and moderate HL using different automated speech-in-noise tests that may be delivered via web or smartphone.

5 Conclusions

In this study we assessed, for the first time, the ability of univariate and multivariate classifiers to identify mild and moderate HL in unscreened adults using a recently validated speech-in-noise test, the WHISPER test. The results showed that the features with highest performance in identifying HL were different between mild and moderate HL. Moreover, results showed that the performance of multivariate classifiers using the full set of available features was better than that of the best-performing univariate classifiers, reaching an accuracy equal to 0.82 and 0.87 for mild and moderate HL, respectively. The results of this study are encouraging and suggest that mild and moderate HL may be discriminated using a small set of features extracted from an automated speech-in-noise screening test, laying the ground for the development of future self-administered speech-in-noise tests viable for screening hearing and cognitive function at a distance and potentially able to provide specific recommendations based on the degree of HL. Access to a mobile application that in a few minutes can give a stratified indication on the degree of HL, considering not only the SRT but a broader picture of the subject, could lead indeed to important benefits to individuals at risk of HL, who can quickly assess their hearing, with improved accuracy as multivariate approaches can help overcome limitations due to well-known mismatch between PTA and SRT in adults.

Acknowledgements. This research work was partially supported by Capita Foundation (project WHISPER, Widespread Hearing Impairment Screening and PrEvention of Risk, 2020 Auditory Research Grant). The authors would like to thank the Lions Clubs International and Associazione La Rotonda, Baranzate (MI) for their contribution in the organization and management of hearing screening and awareness initiatives. The authors are also grateful to all the students who contributed to data collection and to Marta Lenatti and Marco Zanet who contributed to the development of the WHISPER platform.

References

1. Swanepoel, D.W.: eHealth technologies enable more accessible hearing care. In: Seminars in Hearing, vol. 41, no. 02, pp. 133–140 (2020)
2. Paglialonga, A.: eHealth and mHealth for audiologic rehabilitation. In: Montano, J.J., Spitzer, J.B. (eds.) Adult Audiologic Rehabilitation, 3rd edn. Plural Publishing, San Diego (2020)
3. Paglialonga, A., Cleveland Nielsen, A., Ingo, E., Barr, C., Laplante-Lévesque, A.: eHealth and the hearing aid adult patient journey: a state-of-the-art review. BioMed. Eng. Online **17**, 101 (2018). https://doi.org/10.1186/s12938-018-0531-3
4. Paglialonga, A., Tognola, G., Pinciroli, F.: Apps for hearing science and care. Am. J. Audiol. **24**(3), 293–298 (2015). https://doi.org/10.1044/2015_AJA-14-0093
5. Bright, T., Pallawela, D.: Validated smartphone-based apps for ear and hearing assessments: a review. JMIR Rehabil. Assist. Tech. **3**(2), e13 (2016)
6. Davis, A., Smith, P., Ferguson, M., Stephens, D., Gianopoulos, I.: Acceptability, benefit and costs of early screening for hearing disability: a study of potential screening tests and models. Health Technol. Assess. **11**(42), 1–294 (2007)
7. Feltner, C., Wallace, I.F., Kistler, C.E., Coker-Schwimmer, M., Jonas, D.E.: Screening for hearing loss in older adults. JAMA **325**(12), 1202 (2021)
8. Leensen, M.C., de Laat, J.A., Dreschler, W.A.: Speech-in-noise screening tests by Internet, Part 1: test evaluation for noise-induced hearing loss identification. Int. J. Audiol. **50**(11), 823–834 (2011)
9. Smits, C., Kapteyn, T.S., Houtgast, T.: Development and validation of an automatic speech-in-noise screening test by telephone. Int. J. Audiol. **43**(1), 15–28 (2004)
10. Paglialonga, A., Grandori, F., Tognola, G.: Using the speech understanding in noise (SUN) test for adult hearing screening. Am. J. Audiol. **22**(1), 171–174 (2013). https://doi.org/10.1044/1059-0889(2012/12-0055)
11. Paglialonga, A., Tognola, G., Grandori, F.: A user operated test of suprathreshold acuity in noise for adult hearing screening: the SUN (speech understanding in noise) test. Comput. Biol. Med. **52**, 66–72 (2014). https://doi.org/10.1016/j.compbiomed.2014.06.012
12. Paglialonga, A., Polo, E.M., Zanet, M., Rocco, G., van Waterschoot, T., Barbieri, R.: An automated speech-in-noise test for remote testing: development and preliminary evaluation. Am. J. Audiol. **29**(3S), 564–576 (2020). https://doi.org/10.1044/2020_AJA-19-00071

13. Polo, E.M., Zanet, M., Lenatti, M., van Waterschoot, T., Barbieri, R., Paglialonga, A.: Development and evaluation of a novel method for adult hearing screening: towards a dedicated smartphone app. In: Goleva, R., Garcia, N.R.d.C., Pires, I.M. (eds) HealthyIoT 2020. LNICST, vol. 360, pp. 3–19. Springer, Cham (2021). https://doi.org/10.1007/978-3-030-69963-5_1

14. Zanet, M., Polo, E.M., Rocco, G., Paglialonga, A., Barbieri, R.: Development and preliminary evaluation of a novel adaptive staircase procedure for automated speech-in-noise testing. In: Proceedings of the 41st Annual International Conference of the IEEE Engineering in Medicine and Biology Society (EMBC) (2019). https://doi.org/10.1109/EMBC.2019.8857492

15. Zanet, M., et al.: Evaluation of a novel speech-in-noise test for hearing screening: classification performance and transducers characteristics. IEEE J. Biomed. Health Inf. 25(12), 4300–4307 (2021). https://doi.org/10.1109/JBHI.2021.3100368

16. Paglialonga, A., et al.: WHISPER (widespread hearing impairment screening and prevention of risk): a new platform for early identification of hearing impairment and cognitive decline. In: Hearing Across the Lifespan Conference (HEAL), Cernobbio, Italy, 16–18 June 2022

17. Lenatti, M., Moreno-Sánchez, P.A., Polo, E.M., Mollura, M., Barbieri, R., Paglialonga, A.: Evaluation of machine learning algorithms and explainability techniques to detect hearing loss from a speech-in-noise screening test. Am. J. Audiol. 31(3S), 961–979 (2022). https://doi.org/10.1044/2022_AJA-21-00194

18. Humes, L.E.: Understanding the speech-understanding problems of older adults. Am. J. Audiol. 22(2), 303–305 (2013)

19. Killion, M.C., Niquette, P.A.: What can the pure-tone audiogram tell us about a patient's SNR loss? Hear. J. 53(3), 46–48 (2000)

20. Nuesse, T., Steenken, R., Neher, T., Holube, I.: Exploring the link between cognitive abilities and speech recognition in the elderly under different listening conditions. Front. Psychol. 9, 678 (2018)

21. Polo, E.M., Zanet, M., Paglialonga, A., Barbieri, R.: Preliminary evaluation of a novel language independent speech-in-noise test for adult hearing screening. In: Jarm, T., Cvetkoska, A., Mahnič-Kalamiza, S., Miklavcic, D. (eds.) EMBEC 2020. IFMBE Proceedings, vol. 80, pp. 976–983. Springer, Cham (2021). https://doi.org/10.1007/978-3-030-64610-3_109

22. World Health Organization, Deafness and hearing loss. https://www.who.int/news-room/fact-sheets/detail/deafness-and-hearing-loss. Accessed 24 Sept 2022

23. World Health Organization, World report on hearing. https://www.who.int/publications/i/item/world-report-on-hearing. Accessed 24 Sept 2022

24. US Preventive Services Task Force. Screening for Hearing Loss in Older Adults: US Preventive Services Task Force Recommendation Statement. JAMA 325(12), 1196–1201 (2021)

25. Zurek, P., Delhorne, L.A.:Consonant reception in noise by listeners with mild and moderate sensorineural hearing impairment. J. Acoust. Soc. Am. 82(5), 1548–1559 (1987)

26. Summers, V., Makashay, M.J., Theodoroff, S.M., Leek, M.R.: Suprathreshold auditory processing and speech perception in noise: hearing-impaired and normal-hearing listeners. J. Am. Acad. Audiol. 24(4), 274–292 (2010)

27. Füllgrabe, C., Moore, B.C.J., Stone, M.A.: Age-group differences in speech identification despite matched audiometrically normal hearing: Contributions from auditory temporal processing and cognition. Front. Aging Neurosci. 6, 347 (2015)

28. Smith, S.L., Pichora-Fuller, M.K.: Associations between speech understanding and auditory and visual tests of erbal working memory: effects of linguistic complexity, task, age, and hearing loss. Front. Psychol. 6, 1394 (2015)

29. Watson, C.S., Kidd, G.R., Miller, J.D., Smits, C., Humes, L.E.: Telephone screening tests for functionally impaired hearing: current use in seven countries and development of a U.S. version. J. Am. Acad. Audiol. 23(10), 757–767 (2012)

30. Armstrong, N.M., Oosterloo, B.C., Croll, P.H., Ikram, M.A., Goedegebure, A.: Discrimination of degrees of auditory performance from the digits-in-noise test based on hearing status, Int. J. Audiol. **59**(12), 897–904 (2020)

31. Ooster, J., Krueger, M., Bach, J.-H., Wagener, K.C., Kollmeier, B., Meyer, B.T.: Speech audiometry at home: automated listening tests via smart speakers with normal-hearing and hearing-impaired listeners. Trends Hear **24** (2020)

32. Stevens, G., Flaxman, S., Brunskill, E., Mascarenhas, M., Mathers, C.D., Finucane, M.: Global burden of disease hearing loss expert group: global and regional hearing impairment prevalence: an analysis of 42 studies in 29 countries. Eur. J. Pub. Health **23**(1), 146–152 (2013)

A Preliminary Prototype of Smart Healthcare Modular System for Cardiovascular Diseases Remote Monitoring

Valentina Di Pinto[✉][iD], Federico Tramarin[iD], and Luigi Rovati[iD]

Department of Engineering "Enzo Ferrari", University of Modena and Reggio Emilia, Modena, Italy
{valentina.dipinto,federico.tramarin,luigi.rovati}@unimore.it

Abstract. According to the World Health Organization (WHO), about 17.9 millions people per year die from cardiovascular diseases (CVDs), representing more than 32% of all deaths recorded worldwide. Moreover, focusing on the European Society of Cardiology (ESC) member countries, CVDs remain the most common cause of death. Additionally, the worldwide pandemic situation has further underlined the necessity of remote health monitoring systems, aiming at remotely supervising patients by clinicians, able to analyse and record a selected set of parameters with high accuracy levels and promptly identify significant events. In this scenario, this work aims to propose a reconfigurable preliminary prototype of Smart Healthcare Modular System (SHeMS), which combines modularity and real-time signal analysis, leveraging on sensor fusion and Internet of Things technologies. The architecture of the system, as well as the selected main components will be presented, together with the rationale for the development of the whole system. The current evolution of the project has focused particularly on the accurate measurement of the electrocardiographic (ECG) signal, considered the most critical vital parameter for remote monitoring. Besides, the presented ongoing activity is devoted to the implementation of other significant modules, like SpO2, blood pressure, temperature, vocal messages, to enhance monitoring capabilities and increase the detection accuracy of critical events.

Keywords: Remote Health Monitoring · Modular System · Cardiovascular Diseases

1 Introduction

According to the World Health Organization (WHO), about 17.9 million people die per year from to cardiovascular diseases (CVDs). This is more than 32% of all the deaths recorded worldwide, with more than 85% of these deaths caused by heart attacks and strokes, sub-categories of CVDs [1]. Furthermore, the European Society of Cardiology (ESC) reports frightening data related to

S. Spinsante et al. (Eds.): HealthyIoT 2022, LNICST 456, pp. 93–107, 2023.
https://doi.org/10.1007/978-3-031-28663-6_8

CVDs-caused worldwide deaths. As [14] states, CVDs remain the most common cause of death within the ESC member countries, exceeding the number of cancer deaths for both sexes. These data underline the importance of patients' continuous health monitoring, especially for the case of heart failures (HF).

In addition, the worldwide pandemic of Covid-19 has shed light on the critical importance that a new generation of remote health monitoring systems are available. These systems should enable physicians and clinicians to effectively supervise patients remotely, with patients being in their home premises. This is already partially possible, but most of the available systems are non-real-time, providing data in batches once or twice a day, and require both a mobile private and carrier-operated connection, and an access to a private cloud operated by the system manufacturer. These last are high-cost facilities for the healthcare system, and does not allow a full control of the monitoring parameters and periods. Remote monitoring systems should instead support for a continuous and real-time feed of data, measured with the help of potentially wearable devices, able both to analyze and record a selected set of vital parameters, with clinical accuracy levels, and to promptly identify significant events, possibly by means of Artificial Intelligence (AI) algorithms. In this way, the need for hospitalizations would significantly decrease, consequently increasing resource availability for major emergencies as well as reducing the patients' waiting time.

In light of the previous considerations, a novel concept of remote healthcare device can be devised, which may leverages on a sensor fusion approach to enhance analysis capabilities and accuracy, and which is able to provide a continuous and real-time signal analysis. In this paper, the preliminary design of a Smart Healthcare Modular System (SHeMS) is hence proposed, based on a modular paradigm and Internet of Thing (IoT) technologies to enhance both customization and availability of services almost everywhere, and free from carrier-operated services. Modularity is a characterizing feature, allowing the system to be composed around of and adapting to the specific disease and needs of each patient, realizing an interesting reality merging home treatment and care. SHeMS has been devised to provide a seamless, real-time and bi-directional relationship between patients and clinicians, also allowing remote diagnosis, reconfigurability and sensors calibration.

To this goal, the description of this remote monitoring system (SHeMS) prototype is provided where a central unit, hosting the main computing and IoT capabilities, is a gateway for secondary specialized sensing elements. Some of the considered sensing units could be possibly worn by patients, thus directly acquiring and sending to the main computing unit the signals representing relevant vital parameters. The considered vital signs can be related to heart rate (HR), arterial oxygen saturation (SpO2), blood pressure, body temperature and dehydration. Thanks to the modularity of the SHeMS system, additional sensing units could possibly be inserted, e.g. glycemic sensors for diabetic patients and posture sensors. Auxiliary units can be also employed, in order to both test the patient's cognitive competence, through vocal messages, or to simply assist the patient himself/herself and check for some eventual feedback.

This article is organized as follows. First, an introduction and explanation of the vital parameters to investigate will be presented in Sect. 2. Then, in Sect. 3, the needed general specifications will be provided, together with the discussion about the actually employed components. The employed communication protocol is briefly explained in Sect. 3.4, whereas the currently developed software is discussed in Sect. 3.5. Furthermore, a discussion about employed algorithm for the ECG signal manipulation and peaks detection is carried out in Sect. 4, with an emphasis on the future works the authors are committed to. Finally, the most relevant conclusions will be provided in Sect. 5.

2   Vital Parameters of Interest

In order to realize the modular system introduced in Sect. 1, it is necessary to investigate the main vital parameters that should be common for each patient, independently of the clinical history of each subject. The electrocardiographic signal analysis, namely ECG, through the electrocardiogram is the most common test to diagnose CVDs in hospitals [4], thus it is the most important parameter to be investigated. Indeed, through some signal processing algorithms, it also allows to compute the heart rate, another important indicator for CVDs diagnosis. The ECG signal, whose trace is represented in Fig. 1 is constituted by three main components, or complexes:

- P waves;
- QRS-complex;
- T waves.

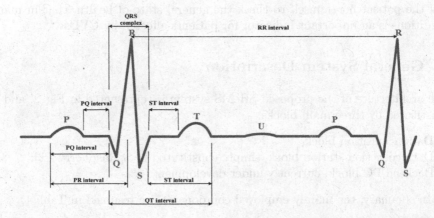

Fig. 1. ECG signal trace

P-waves, in physiological conditions, alternate periodically. More in detail, they represents the atrium depolarization, thus occurring for first and has a general duration of about 110 ms [8]. After P wave, the QRS-complex is registered. It is constituted by three different peaks (namely, Q, R, S) and represents the depolarization of the ventricle, defining the onset of the ventricular contraction. Its normal duration ranges about 60 ms−100 ms [13] and it is the easiest complex to identify, due to its amplitude with respect to the other waves. The last complex that is worth mentioning is the T wave, thus the representation of the ventricle repolarization [7]. Its duration in physiological conditions is about 100 ms−250 ms [9]. After describing the ECG signal components it is possible to conclude that the spectral content of the ECG signal belongs to the low frequencies range (approximately 0.5 Hz−150 Hz). Foreseeing the useful signal contributes, the highest frequency contribute is contained into the QRS-complex. The lowest frequency contribute is instead contained into the P and T waves, even though they are important indicators of many CVDs. From the analysis of the ECG peaks and characteristics it is possible to detect heart anomalies, together with the heart rate. From the heart rate, another parameter of interest, it is possible to extract the heart rate variability (HRV), that records the beat-to-beat variations of HR, and the intervals between R-R peaks intervals (QRS-complexes) [10]. Another important parameter strictly related to CVDs and other relevant diseases is the blood pressure, namely BP (both systolic and diastolic). As [16] states, there is a strong and significant association between BP and risk of CVDs and this relation is independent of other risk factors for CVDs (e.g. age, gender, body weight). For example, hypertension is considered the leading preventable risk factor for both CVDs and all-cause mortality in developing countries. Blood oxygen saturation (SpO2) and temperature are two additional parameters to be taken into account since they allow the clinician and the patient her/himself to check the general state of health, that in many conditions is an important indicator for patients affected by CVDs.

3   General System Description

The architecture of the proposed SHeMS system is represented in Fig. 2, and is constituted by three main blocks:

- Data acquisition block;
- Data collection station block, simply constituted by a Raspberry Pi3;
- Backend PC block, currently under development.

In summary, the mainly employed components are resumed in Table 1.

3.1   Data Acquisition Block

An important requirement for this block is to be lightweight and sufficiently small, since it has to be worn by the subject. Its simplified schematic is represented in Fig. 3, where a microcontroller based on the ESP32 architecture is

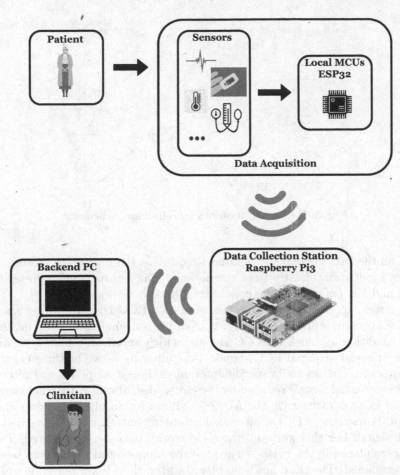

Fig. 2. SHeMS general architecture

Table 1. Employed components

Component Type	Component Name	Role	Communication Way
Microcontroller	ESP32 - WROOM32	Data acquisition	Serial with sensor, MQTT with data collection station
Processing unit	Raspberry Pi 3	Data collection station	MQTT with data acquisition block
Sensor	AD8232	Sensing unit as a part of data acquisition block	Serial with microcontroller

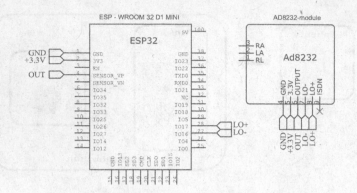

Fig. 3. Data acquisition block preliminary schematic

shown on the left, whereas the rightmost module is the measuring sensor, which receives input data directly from the patient. The sensing unit represented in Figs. 2 and 3 is only one of the possible employable devices.

In particular, the current choice has been on a ECG-trace recording based on the AD8232 chip, represented in Fig. 4a [2]. This is a small and cheap integrated signal conditioning block for ECG signals, which specifically allows to manipulate single-lead acquired ECG signals, thus allowing a two or three electrodes configuration. Thanks to its specific internal design, it amplifies and filters the small biopotential signals received by the electrodes, also in noisy conditions. As reported in its datasheet [2], the AD82838 allows for an ultralow power analog-to- digital converter (ADC) or an embedded microcontroller to easily acquire the output signal. For this work, all three electrodes have been employed. Two of them were placed in the wrists, to acquire the biopotential that has to be effectively examined. The third has been placed in the right lower pelvis, in order to reduce the common-mode interference [15].

Together with the AD8232, the data acquisition block is constituted by a microcontroller directly connected to the sensing unit. In this case, an ESP32-WROOM-32 [6] has been employed, which is represented in Fig. 4b. This module presents some significant advantages, the main being:

– Cheapness;
– Compact size and low weight;
– Built-in IoT/network support;
– Printed on board antenna;
– Dual-core possible operation.

One of the most attracting feature of the chosen computing module is its intrinsic support for data transmission over a Wi-Fi network. This is an ideal feature for this project, since the data acquired from connected sensors can be previously stored in a convenient format, and then sent to a data collection unit, or central gateway, the second block of SHeMS, which resides in the surroundings of the

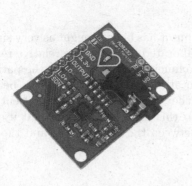   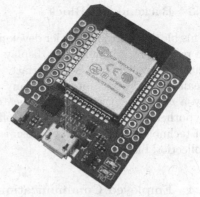

(a) AD8232 single-lead heart rate monitor   (b) ESP WROOM 32 board

Fig. 4. Components currently employed in the data acquisition block

patient, typically within the same building. This will allows module-to-module communications without the need for further network support, and also might possibly exploit already existent Wi-Fi networks. Furthermore, an extremely interesting feature is the presence of two cores, since due to the high amount of data to be acquire and then transmitted, it is hence possible to split the workload in parallel over the two cores, with one continuously managing the sensing units for data acquisition, and the other one instead devoted only to the management of the network interface.

It is worth mentioning that although this work will only briefly discuss the simulation viewpoint in Sect. 4, between the AD8232 and the ESP32 control unit a filtering stage for noise suppression has been designed. In particular, the main noise sources are [5]:

- Baseline wander, caused by different factors, such as respiration, body movements, poor skin-electrode contact;
- Powerline interference;
- Muscle artifacts.

3.2 Data Collection Block

This block is mainly constituted by a Raspberry Pi3 located in the same building of the data acquisition block, as previously mentioned in Sect. 3.1. Basically, it should continuously acquire data, received from the data acquisition station, for a quite long amount of time (e.g. a couple of hours), to let the clinician check the patient health status. After the data collection, it simply elaborates it, following the logic briefly presented in Sect. 4. So far, the latter has been simulated on Matlab, thus not guaranteeing sequentiality between data acquisition and elaboration. The authors are committed to reproduce the same algorithm in another programming language, in order to let Raspberry Pi3 do the final data elaboration.

3.3   Backend PC Block

This block is currently under development but it has been thought as very simple. In particular, it should only display the elaborated data and the relative results, thus merely being a User Interface for the clinician to finally check the patient's health status and not having any computational power. Needing to be used by a clinician, it will not be located in the surroundings of the patient but, hypothetically, in the clinician's office. To this aim, the authors will use Wi-Fi technology for the data transmission between the backend PC and the data collection block.

3.4   Employed Communication Protocol

After introducing the general system architecture, it is worth spending some words about the communication protocol stack chosen for data exchange over Wi-Fi, namely MQTT (Message Queue Telemetry Transport).

This is a widespread, simple and lightweight publish/subscribe communication protocol, very interesting for IoT applications (employed for instance in healthcare, energy and utilities, social networking [12]), especially for the case of limited-capabilities smart devices [11], as those employed in this work. It relies on the TCP/IP classic protocol stack, and in particular it typically exploits TCP at the transport layer to ensure the needed reliability. At the same time MQTT is lightweight in that it defines control messages with a very low overhead: these require just a 2 Bytes fixed header, which can be possibly expanded, followed directly by the user payload.

At the base of the MQTT protocol there is a Publish/Subscribe model [12]. Here, the *Publisher* publishes messages to the *Broker*, while the *Subscriber* subscribes to the so-called *topics*, that can be basically considered message subjects. When subscribing to particular *topics*, the *Subscriber* is able to receive every message published to the latter ones. The architecture of an MQTT network involves the entities *Client* and *Broker*. More in detail, as it is possible to see in Fig. 5, the *Client* can be both a *Publisher* or *Subscriber* and is in charge of establishing the network connection to the *Broker*. A client, once connected, can publish messages relevant to a specific subject, subscribe to other subjects for receiving messages, unsubscribe to subscribed subjects, and detach from the *Broker* [12]. The *Broker* in turn receives all the messages from the *Client*, thus being able to decide whether to accept or not *Client* requests. Furthermore, it can receive published messages by the users, process different requests like *Subscribe* and *Unsubscribe* from the users and send the latter to the users.

MQTT supports three levels of Quality of Service (QoS):

- QoS0: the message is sent at most once, thus not necessarily guaranteeing the message delivery;
- QoS1: the message is sent at least once;
- QoS2: through 4-ways handshaking, the message is sent once.

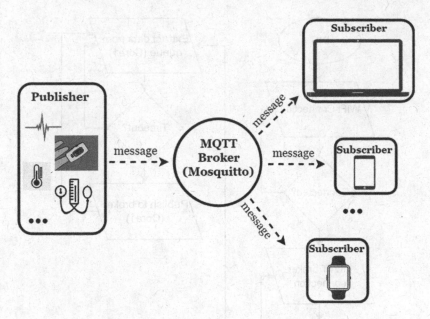

Fig. 5. MQTT protocol architecture

The selection of the QoS level depends on the specific application. In this case, QoS0 has been preliminarily employed, since it represents the option with the lower cost in terms of data transfer volume. Additionally, the connection between the *Publisher* (in this case, the ESP32 module) and the *Broker* (with reference to Fig. 2, the Raspberry Pi3 board) was considered reliable, also thanks to the operation environment, considered pretty close to the real future application of the system (at the patient's home). Clearly, the intended application aims at highly reliable acquisition of vital parameters, therefore the QoS level choice will be further investigated in next project steps.

3.5 Developed Software

In this Section, the developed software for the correct operation of each block will be presented. In particular, the following algorithms will be briefly discussed:

- MQTT *Publisher-Broker* data exchange and connection (*Publisher* side);
- Acquired ECG signal manipulation for peaks detection.

The code relative to the MQTT *Publisher-Broker* connection, at *Broker* side is not discussed due to its simplicity. Indeed, it simply initially checks whether

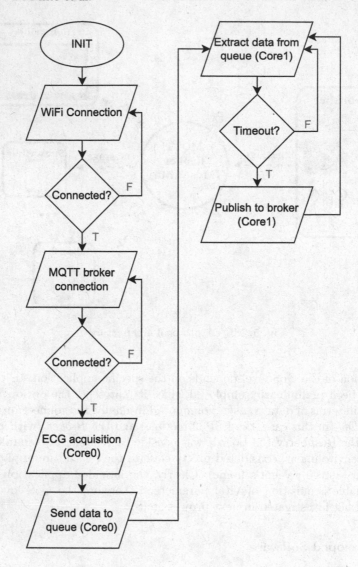

Fig. 6. Flowchart for the MQTT *Publisher-Broker* data exchange and connection (*Publisher* side)

the *Broker*, that is the Raspberry Pi3, is connected to the *Publisher*, that is the ESP32. Then, it continuously acquires the data received by the *Publisher* and saves the latter into a text file. The data acquisition and the connection can be stopped in any moment.

3.6   MQTT *Publisher-Broker* Data Exchange and Connection (*Publisher* Side)

In order to better understand the working principle under this algorithm, a flowchart is represented in Fig. 6. After establishing the Wi-Fi connection, the connection to the Mosquitto *Broker* is performed, through the employment of a readily available library, namely the PubSubClient library. Nevertheless, its usage will be reviewed in future implementation, since it currently presents some limitations in terms of choice of the QoS level, although at the moment the chosen QoS0 level is supported without issues.

Then, two parallel tasks (threads) are executed over the two cores of the ESP32 microcontroller. In particular, the first task is performed by Core0, and is relevant to the acquisition of the ECG signal measurements. The sampling rate of the acquisition process has been set to $f_s = 720$ Hz, where each sample is represented by a 4 Bytes floating point data. These measurements are immediately stored within a suitably defined FIFO queue whose size is 3 KB, thus allowing for a maximum storage of 750 samples. In parallel, the second task is run over Core1, and its main duties are the extraction of new samples from the queue, the encapsulation within an MQTT control message and the subsequent transmission over Wi-Fi. Specifically, samples extraction is performed over a period of 1 s (i.e. 720 samples are collected) with the consequent creation of a payload of 2880 Bytes for the MQTT message. Once the message is ready, Core1 initiates an immediate transmission over the Wi-Fi link, to publish the new information message to the *Broker*. The chosen parameters, i.e. the queue size and the transmission period, have been defined to ensure, on the one hand to decrease the Wi-Fi link usage as much as possible, to improve energy efficiency, trading off with the payload length to avoid data loss over the Wi-Fi link. On the other hand, such parameters ensure a continuous acquisition from the measurement ADC.

4   Algorithm for ECG Signal Manipulation and Peaks Detection: Preliminary Results

In this section, the first preliminary results obtained for the ECG signal acquisition are presented. In particular, at first the signal conditioning technique is described. Then, this is applied to the signals acquired by means of the aforementioned sensor (i.e. the AD8232), which is connected to the ESP32 module, which in turn encapsulates them into MQTT control messages sent over wireless to the Raspberry Pi3 *Broker*.

As it is possible to see in Fig. 7, after acquiring the data from the *Broker* and saving it to a text file, a preprocessing has been carried out. As stated in Sect. 3.1, this filtering stage is a simulation of the analog filtering stages that will be introduced in the data acquisition block, in order to manage the noise and interference issues. As previously introduced in Sect. 2, the ECG signal frequencies of interest range from 0.5 Hz to approximately 150 Hz.

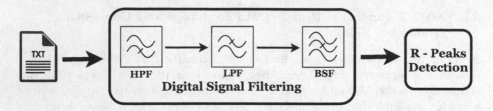

Fig. 7. Signal processing block diagram

Therefore, at first a high pass filter (HPF) with a cut-off frequency of $f_1 = 0.5\,$Hz has been implemented, followed by a low pass filter (LPF) whose cut-off frequency is set at $f_2 = 150\,$Hz. Then, a band-stop filter (BSF) with $f_3 = 50\,$Hz center frequency has been applied, in order to address the powerline interference issue. Besides the filtering stage, other secondary signal processing operations have been programmatically performed, like signals resampling at $f_s = 720\,$Hz and successive normalization to maximum. Subsequently, a pair of derivative filters and max filtering were employed for peaks detection, following the approach suggested in [3]. The derivative and max filters were applied on windows of $W = 4000\,$samples with a sliding window of size $S = 3200\,$samples, thus with an overlap between windows of $\frac{1}{5}W$.

The result can be appreciated in Figs. 8 and 9, for signals acquired with a duration of 60 s. As stated in Sect. 3.1, the electrodes in charge of the ECG-acquisition were positioned in correspondence of the wrists and the third electrode was positioned in the right lower pelvis. Foreseeing the ECG signal represented in Fig. 8, the patient did not carry out very fast movements but simply stood up and down, moved the arms and hands and slowly walked. The R-peaks are all successfully detected, albeit also two P-wave peaks have been also marked. In order to overcome this issue, a comparison algorithm is being developed.

The compared signals are the one resulting from the application of the algorithm of [3] and a signal resulting from a band-pass filter, to which an envelope signal has been applied. In this way the missing R-peaks can be inserted and the erroneously detected P-wave peaks can be removed. The signal presented in Fig. 9 is instead characterized by only noise, thus the patient moved very fast the wrists, thus worsening the skin-electrodes contact surface, stood up and down very rapidly and without caring about the presence of the right lower pelvis-positioned electrode, so as to dirty the acquired signal trace as much as possible.

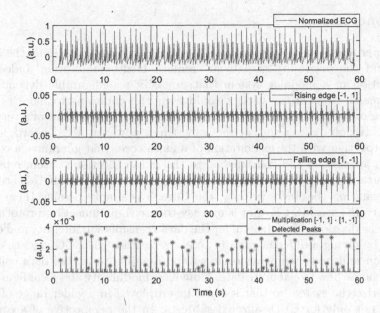

Fig. 8. R-peak detection algorithm for a signal characterized by a low-noise level. The patient stood up and down quite slowly and did some steps calmly

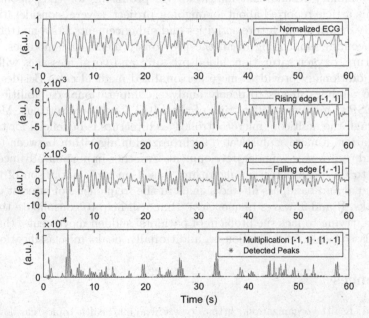

Fig. 9. R-peak detection algorithm for a signal characterized by only noise. As it is possible to notice, no R-peaks have been detected by the algorithm. The patient carried out very fast movements, trying to be as much agitated as possible

5   Conclusions

This paper addressed a very hot research topic, further underlining the importance and the possibility of patients' remote health monitoring. Indeed, the introduction of a modular system that is easily reconfigurable depending on the clinical history of the patient could help the clinicians to more precisely provide more accurate diagnosis to the patients. The employment of a very compact, lightweight, cheap and, at the same time, powerful MCU board, such as ESP32, together with the exploitation of its two cores that guarantee a continuous data acquisition and transmission to the data collection station, represents an important point for this research. While the Core 0 of the MCU is acquiring data, basing on the Tasks priority, the Core 1 is simply passing them to the Raspberry Pi3 via MQTT, that is an easy-to-use communication protocol. The code Tasks division is very helpful for the data transmission integrity and clarity. Indeed, by giving a different priority to each Task for the ECG signals, oxygen saturation and body temperature, it will be possible to let the data collection station choose how to elaborate data. Moreover, modularity and reconfigurability characterize the system so that it could be employed in a wider range of applications, not only for CVDs-affected subjects. In the perspective of a complete development of the described system, namely SHeMS, the authors presented some preliminary results that appear to be promising for the ongoing work. While this article reported about an ongoing project, several considerations can be already drawn about future activities and enhancements. As a matter of fact, the forthcoming embedding of all the previously mentioned modules, such as temperature, oxygen saturation, blood pressure and vocal messages will clearly help to additionally provide a more personalized medical care. Besides, inserting these modules means to deeply analyze computational capabilities of the chosen ESP32 microcontrollers, and of the MQTT protocol settings. Moreover, even though the multicore microcontroller architecture is beneficial for this type of application, a more sophisticated sychronization algorithm between the *Publisher* and the *Broker* is under development. Another important advancement is relevant to the peak detection algorithm, based on the comparison of the processed signal and bandpass filtered signals in the frequencies of interest (relative to R-peaks, P and T waves frequencies), that will help to consolidate the peaks detection, trying to face the problem of patients' sudden movements, that could imply missed peaks' classification or, additionally, peaks misclassification.

References

1. World health organization. https://www.who.int/health-topics/cardiovascular-diseases
2. Analog devices: AD8232 (3 2020). https://www.analog.com/media/en/technical-documentation/data-sheets/ad8232.pdf
3. Bae, T.W., Kwon, K.K.: Efficient real-time R and QRS detection method using a pair of derivative filters and max filter for portable ECG device. Appl. Sci. 9(19), 4128 (2019). https://doi.org/10.3390/app9194128

4. Bai, B., Zhao, Y., Chen, X., Chen, Y., Luo, Z.: A smart portable ECG monitoring system with high precision and low power consumption. J. Intell. Fuzzy Syst. **41**, 1–11 (2021). https://doi.org/10.3233/JIFS-189715

5. Chatterjee, S., Thakur, R.S., Yadav, R.N., Gupta, L., Raghuvanshi, D.K.: Review of noise removal techniques in ECG signals. IET Signal Proc. **14**(9), 569–590 (2020). https://doi.org/10.1049/iet-spr.2020.0104

6. Espressif Systems: ESP32 (3 2022), v. 3.8. https://www.espressif.com/sites/default/files/documentation/esp32-datasheet-en.pdf

7. Fong, S., et al.: Electrocardiogram signal classification in the diagnosis of heart disease based on rbf neural network. Comput. Math. Methods Med. (2022). https://doi.org/10.1155/2022/9251225

8. Kahyaoglu, M., et al.: The usefulness of morphology-voltage-p wave duration ECG score for predicting early left atrial dysfunction in hypertensive patients. Clin. Exper. Hyper. **43**(6), 572–578 (2021). https://doi.org/10.1080/10641963.2021.1916945. pMID: 33866872

9. Madeiro, J., Cortez, P., Monteiro, J., Rodrigues, P.: Mathematical modeling of t-wave and p-wave: a robust alternative for detecting and delineating those waveforms, pp. 141–167 (2018). https://doi.org/10.1016/B978-0-12-814035-2.00012-8

10. Owens, A.P.: The role of heart rate variability in the future of remote digital biomarkers. Front. Neurosci. **14**, 582145 (2020). https://doi.org/10.3389/fnins.2020.582145. https://www.frontiersin.org/articles/10.3389/fnins.2020.582145

11. Sahmi, I., Mazri, T., Hmina, N.: A comparative study of MQTT with the applications protocols of IoT. ResearchGate (2018). https://www.researchgate.net/publication/329644161. A-comparative-study-of-MQTT-with-the-Applications-Protocols-of-IoT

12. Soni, D., Makwana, A.: A survey on MQTT: a protocol of internet of things (IoT) (2017)

13. Tereshchenko, L., Josephson, M.: Frequency content and characteristics of ventricular conduction. J. Electrocardiol. **48**, 933–937 (2015). https://doi.org/10.1016/j.jelectrocard.2015.08.034

14. Timmis, A., et al.: European society of cardiology: cardiovascular disease statistics 2021. Eur. Heart J. **43**(8), 716–799 (2022). https://doi.org/10.1093/eurheartj/ehab892

15. do Vale Madeiro, J.P., Cortez, P.C., da Silva Monteiro Filho, J.M., Brayner, A.R.A.: Developments and applications for ECG signal processing. Elsevier, Academic Press (2019). https://doi.org/10.1016/C2017-0-01102-3

16. Wang, H., et al.: Blood pressure, body mass index and risk of cardiovascular disease in Chinese men and women. BMC Public Health **10**, 189 (2010). https://doi.org/10.1186/1471-2458-10-189

Gender Classification Using nonstandard ECG Signals - A Conceptual Framework of Implementation

Henriques Zacarias[1,2]([⊠]) [iD], Virginie Felizardo[1,2] [iD], Leonice Souza-Pereira[1,2] [iD], André Pinho[1,2], Susana Ramos[2], Mehran Pourvahab[2] [iD], Nuno Garcia[1,2] [iD], and Nuno Pombo[1,2] [iD]

[1] Instituto de Telecomunicações, Covilhã, Portugal
henriques.zacarias@ubi.pt
[2] ALLab - Assisted Living Computing and Telecommunications Laboratory, Universidade da Beira Interior, Covilhã, Portugal
https://www.it.pt/ITSites/Index/6

Abstract. This paper presents a comparison of nine models for gender identification using nonstandard ECG signal. Methods: QRS features, QT interval, RR interval, HRV features and HR were extracted from three minutes of 40 ECG's (from 24 female and 16 males) available at ALLab dataset and 108 ECG's (from 52 female and 56 males) available at CYBHi dataset. Models were developed using Decision tree, SVM, kNN, Boosted tree, Bagged tree, Subspace kNN, Subspace Discriminant, two majority vote and verified by external validation. Results: The study presented achieved as best results an accuracy of 78% from Boosted tree and 85% from majority vote. Conclusion: The automatic detection of gender by ECG could be very important and improve the development of predictive systems for cardiovascular disease. These classifications are promising due to the use of nonstandard ECG and to the simplicity of extraction of features that potentiated the correct classification

Keywords: Gender classification · nonstandard ECG · Real data · Machine learning

1 Introduction

The use of Electrocardiogram (ECG) signal to establish a person identity is an approach of biometrics by using features of an ECG signal as the inputs to an

This work was partially funded by FCT/MCTES through national funds and co-funded by the FEDER-PT2020 partnership agreement under the project UIDB/50008/2020. This article is based on work from COST Action IC1303-AAPELE-Architectures, Algorithms and Protocols for Enhanced Living Environments and COST Action CA16226-SHELD-ON-Indoor living space improvement: Smart Habitat for the Elderly, supported by COST (European Cooperation in Science and Technology).

S. Spinsante et al. (Eds.): HealthyIoT 2022, LNICST 456, pp. 108–120, 2023.
https://doi.org/10.1007/978-3-031-28663-6_9

identification or authentication system. The feature extraction process results in five major deflection points (labeled P, Q, R, S and T) that combined show the ECG waveform. Besides these features, other ECG features are also used such as time domain features and frequency domain features, e.g., wavelet transform and power spectral density.

There are different types of ECG, depending upon the number of electrodes, such as 1-lead, 2-Lead, 6-Lead, and 12-Lead. The 12-lead ECG has many benefits over other kinds, including a) properly recreating the QRS, ST, and T waveforms, b) giving evidence of P wave and QRS complex morphology that cannot be detected with a single-lead ECG, and c) observing the changes in the ST segment the best. Thus, the 12-lead ECG became the standard electrocardiography [6, 25]. Despite these advantages, nonstandard ECG can be suitable as a screening device for pathological rhythms or as ECG-based biometric system.

Prevention, management and treatment of many diseases do not reflect one of the most important risk factor for the patients, the gender [27]. There are important physiological differences between the two genders which deserve the attention of the scientific community, as to allow more relevance to "gender medicine" based on risk profiles, and to support the development of new predictive algorithms. Some cardiovascular diseases (CVD) have more prevalence in women than men, e.g. angina pectoris and stroke, and inversely coronary heart disease and heart failure have more prevalence in men than women. Gender is an essential, although sometimes overlooked, factor in determining human health. Clinical results, as well as the efficacy and safety of regularly used medications, may be significantly impacted by both sex and gender-related characteristics [15]. Recently, the incorporation of sex and gender views in clinical research and other sectors of adult health has enhanced the understanding of several diseases and produced convincing evidence for a more customized healthcare strategy [19, 28]. Increased awareness of gender-specific differences-in basic and applied research, clinical portrayal, design of treatment regimens and procedures, guidelines, preventive strategies, and public health policies-may improve individualized care, appropriately address the unique needs of genders and sub-populations, and thereby reduce inequities, as well as present and future disease burden at the individual, community, national, and global scales [19, 20]. Despite this, the sex- and gender-informed approach to medicine is a relatively new field based on current research, and it should be incorporated into both preclinical and clinical investigations to comprehend both male and female variations and obtain a fully individualized therapy [20, 26].

Gender classification is a task relatively easy for humans, usually done through visual contact while assessing body shape and size, hair patterns, posture, facial features, clothing, or voice, not in this particular order and subject to cultural and environmental setting. Yet, for an identification system, this task can be a major challenge. In [16] the human gender classification is categorized into appearance and non-appearance approaches. Among the appearance approaches, we found still features, dynamic body features and apparel features, while the non-appearance approaches include biometrics features, bio-signals features and social information. In the last decade, the development of small acquisition devices that allow the collection of bio-signals in different scenarios has gained the attention of the scientific community. Of particular interest to this research, some bio-signals are used for gender classification, such as encephalography (EEG), ECG and deoxyribonucleic acid (DNA) [16].

Gender classification has applications in different fields which stand out: mobile applications and video games, demographic research, commercial development, surveillance systems, Human-Computer Interaction, and healthcare [33].

Relatively to gender differences in ECG signal Kumar et al. [14] concluded that male athletes had significantly greater QRS duration, Q-wave duration, and T wave amplitude and female athletes had a significantly greater QT interval. Xue & Farrell [34] also concluded that QRS duration is higher in men and QT interval is higher in female.

Research works on gender classification systems using ECG is still scarce, and we will briefly detail some of them (Table 1).

Different methods have been proposed previously for gender classification using ECG signals [1,4,7,9,10,12,13,17]. Some works used datasets with 12-lead ECG signals [4,9], but most of works used other configuration more suitable for a context of identification [1,7,10,12]. From ECG feature extraction, time domain (TD), frequency domain (FD), QRS features, heart rate variability (HRV), wavelets transform (WT), power spectral density (PSD) are commonly used, but some works proposed features based on Poincare section [10] or features based on Attractor Reconstruction (AR) [17]. Among the machine learning techniques highlights SVM, decision tree, kNN and CNN.

This paper is focused on the performance comparison of the nine models, three based on individual classifiers, four are ensembles and two models based on consensus decision using majority vote method, for gender identification using an ECG signal.

In the present study, 108 ECG signals (from 52 female and 56 male) are used to train the different models and 40 ECG's have been recorded (from 24 female and 16 male) to validate the models. For feature extraction the QRS features, QT interval, RR interval, heart rate (HR) and other HRV features were considered, and the following seven different classifiers have been trained and tested for gender classification: Decision tree (DT), Support vector machine (SVM), k-nearest neighbors (kNN), Boosted Tree, Bagged Tree, Subspace Bagged Discriminant, Subspace Bagged kNN. Also, we proposed two decision consensus using majority vote to balance out the individual models weaknesses. The remainder of this paper is organized as follows: this paragraph concludes section I, where the goal of the research was announced, and a brief but concise report of the most significant previous research was presented. Section II is limited to the presentation of the datasets used in this work. Section III describes the methodology and section IV presents the results. Discussion of the results follows in section V and section VI concludes this paper.

Table 1. Previous studies

Study(year)	Dataset	Features	Techniques	Results (Acc)
Tripathy et al. (2012) [13]	37 sets of input-output patterns	HRV	LS-SVM (RBF Kernel Function), 12 sets validation	92%
Ergin et al. (2014) [9]	MIT-BIH normal sinus rhythm (5M /13F)	QRS, TD, WT and PSD	C4.5 decision tree	f-score: 98.6%
Lyle et al. (2017) [17]	ecgrdvq database (11F/11 M)	AR and TD	SVM (Leave one-patients data-out validation)	93.1 (AR), 74% (TD)
Cabra et al. (2018) [7]	ECG-ID 308 templates (50%F)	TD	kNN (5-fold validation)	88.0%
Cabra et al. (2018) [7]	CYBHi. 1750 F F 469M Synthetic: 1281 M templates	TD	kNN (30% holdout validation)	95.1%
Attia et al. (2019) [4]	Train 499727 patients, 52%M Test 275056 patients	n/a	CNN (399750 training and 99977 in the internal validation)	90,4%
Goshvarpour & Goshvarpour (2019) [10]	ECG-ID 37 M 42 F	Poincare section-based	SVM (5-fold validation)	93.66%
Khan et al. (2020) [12]	ECG-ID 90 patients (153M and 159 F templates)	TD, FD	Fine decision tree (10-fold validation)	95.2%
Al Alkeem et al. (2021) [1]	ECG-ID: 44M 46F and PTB ECG: 209 M 81 F, 58 virtual patients	QRS	CNN (validation on virtual data)	90.04% (NA) 83.33% (MD) 82.18% (MD and NA) 100% (DA)

M- male; F- female;

2 Data

2.1 ALLAB Dataset

The experimental installation consists of a wireless physiological data acquisition system bioPlux [24] (1000 Hz sampling rate, 12 bits sample size), which is connected to an ECG sensor (Gain: 1000, band-pass: 0.05 Hz–30 Hz, common-mode rejection ratio: 110 dB). According to the ECG lead placement protocol, the three ECG leads were placed in the horizontal plane precordial position (V3, V4, V5). In this study we collected 40 ECGs at rest during 3–5 minutes from 16 male and 24 female, with ages between 18 and 72 years old, with a mean age of 33.09 ± 18.7 years. The collected data is transmitted from the device to a computer using a Bluetooth connection and an application that was provided by the manufacturer [24] recorded the data in a text file organized in a column-formatted manner. The 4th column corresponds to ECG signal (except for three files that the 2nd column corresponds to ECG). This data was collected as part of the research work for the BSc project in Bioengineering, subject "Caracter-ização de género através de um sinal ECG" (in English "Gender Classification through an ECG signal"). The data used in this research is publicly available at the ALLab MediaWiki [2].

The volunteers were informed of the nature and purpose of this research, an Ethics Committee approved the experimental protocol and the subjects signed an informed consent form. The volunteers declared to be healthy and to suffer from no cardiac disease.

2.2   CYBHi Dataset

The Check Your Biosignals Here initiative (CYBHi) dataset [32] is composed of short-term and long-term signals, the data acquisition was made using a bioplux device with a sampling rate of 1000 Hz Hz. The short-term signals were collected for an overall total of 65 participants, where 49 males and 16 females and the average age of 31.1 ± 9.46 years. ECG signals at the hand palms and fingers were recorded.

A set of 63 subjects, 14 males and 49 females, with an average age of 20.68 ± 2.83 years, were available for data acquisition of long-term signals. ECG signals at the fingers were recorded. In both cases, none of the participants reported any health problems.

3   Methodology

The proposed method is composed of a sequence of processing steps: data prepa-ration, feature extraction and classification.

3.1   Data Preparation and Feature Extraction

The ECG signals extracted from the individual data file of each participant are carried out in MATLAB software. The 148 ECGs are analyzed and we opted to use only the first three minutes of each signal (180000 samples). As pre-processing the base line drift and drive direct current (DC) are removed and a Savitzky-Golay filter [30] is used to smooth out some of the noise from the ECGs, due to its ability to smooth ECG without much destroying its original properties [5,11].

The features used in this work can be listed as time domain (TD) features (RR interval, QT interval, QRS complex amplitude and duration), HRV features (SDNN, RMS, NN50 and PNN50) and heart rate.

From the TD feature extraction process results the detection of five deflection points, labeled P, Q, R, S and T waves. The P wave is an upward deflection and appears before the Q wave, depicting a downward deflection. The R wave follows as an upward deflection and the S wave is downward deflected following the R wave. The Q, R and S are successive waves and together create the QRS complex, with a duration 0,08–0,12 s [31], and a quite variable amplitude from lead to lead and from person to person. The T wave is an upward deflection and follows the S wave.

The RR interval (0,6–1 s [8]) is the duration between successive heart beats and the QT interval is the duration between the beginning of the Q wave and the end of the T wave (0,35–0,43 s [31]). The QT interval calculation is dependent of correct detection of the beginning of the Q wave and the end of the T wave. Statistical features have been extracted from the QT intervals, RR intervals, QRS amplitude and duration, and HR. Figure 1 shows an ECG waveform with the associated features labeled.

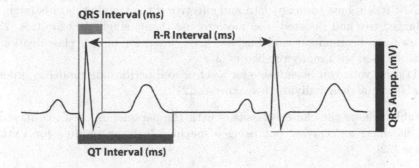

Fig. 1. ECG waveform with the associated features labeled.

Also, we extracted heart rate (HR), the standard deviation of the RR intervals (SDNN), the root mean square of successive differences between RR intervals (rMSSD), the number of times successive heartbeat intervals exceed 50ms (NN50) and the proportion of consecutive RR intervals that differ by more than 50ms (PNN50). Table 2 shows the 24 feature extracted from each subject ECG.

Table 2. Features Extraction.

Features	
QT interval (ms)	Mean, standard deviation, variance, maximum and minimum
RR interval (ms)	Mean, variance, maximum and minimum
Amplitude QRS (mV)	Mean, standard deviation, variance, maximum and minimum
Duration QRS (ms)	Mean, standard deviation, variance, maximum and minimum
HRV	SDNN, rMSSD, NN50, PNN50
HR	Mean

3.2 Classifiers

As the literature on gender classification with ECG is scarce, we have chosen to use several types of classifiers in order to verify which one presents better performances. The choices were made based on their features:

- Decision tree: provides an output easily interpreted by humans, it is fast, but the algorithm is greedy (there is a trade-off here); provides fast prediction but it depends always on the dataset [29].
- SVM: Provides fast predictions for binary classifications, the risk of over fitting is reduced, deliver a unique solution (no local minima), provides the maximum separating margin for a linearly separable dataset (approximation to bound on the test error rate), Kernel trick allows non-linearly separable dataset to may be linearly separable in a higher dimensional space [35].
- kNN: It is robust to noisy data and effective if the training data is large.
- Bagged tree and Boosted tree: more robust than a single decision tree [23].
- Subspace discriminant and Suspace kNN: good for binary classification, it can be used with many predictors [3].
- Majority vote: can be suitable for a set of well performing model in order to balance out their individual weaknesses [21].

Table 3 shows the chosen classifiers with the parameters used in this study. The classifiers are carried out using a machine learning module for Python, sklearn [22].

3.3 Train and Leave-One-Dataset-Out Validation

The dataset used to train the models contains 108 samples, from both short-term and long-term of CYBHi dataset, in which 52 samples are ECGs from females and 56 are ECGs from males. Thus, a 2-class dataset was obtained where each class had ECG features from male (class 1) and female (class 0) subjects. The validation method used is the leave-one-dataset-out using the ALLab dataset that contains 40 samples, in which 24 samples are ECGs from females and 16 are ECGs from males.

Table 3. Classifiers parametrization.

Classifiers	Classifier Type	Classifier Parameters
Decision tree	sklearn.tree.DecisionTreeClassifier	Maximum leaf nodes: 10 Split criterion: entropy Maximum features: auto
SVM	sklearn.svm.SVC	Kernel: rbf Regularization parameter: C=10
kNN	sklearn.neighbors.KNeighborsClassifier	Number of neighbours: 2
Boosted Tree	sklearn.ensemble.AdaBoostClassifier	number of estimators: 400 Learning rate: 0.5 Algorithm: SAMME
Bagged Tree	sklearn.ensemble.AdaBoostClassifier	number of estimators: 30 Maximum features:4 Random state: 4
Subspace Bagged kNN	sklearn.ensemble.BaggingClassifier	Base estimator: KNeighborsClassifier(2) number of estimators: 30 bootstrap=False Maximum features:4
Subspace Bagged Discriminant	sklearn.ensemble.BaggingClassifier	Base estimator: LinearDiscriminantAnalysis(solver='eigen', shrinkage='auto') number of estimators: 10 bootstrap=False Maximum features:4
Majority vote 1	sklearn.ensemble.VotingClassifier	Estimators: Boosted tree, Subspace kNN Voting: hard
Majority vote 2	sklearn.ensemble.VotingClassifier	Estimators: Boosted tree, Subspace kNN, Bagged tree Voting: hard

4   Results

Analysing the results presented in Table 4, it can be seen that different classifiers have different behaviours. In this study, overall, nine classifiers were applied (seven different and two majority votes based on the sevens) in order to detect person gender through ECG signal.

The accuracy and recall are calculated (see Eqs. 1 and 2) with the values extracted from the confusion matrix: True Positive (TP), True Negative (TN), False Positive (FP) and False Negative (FN).

$$Accuracy = \frac{TP + TN}{TP + TN + FP + FN} \tag{1}$$

$$Recall = \frac{TP}{TP + FN} \tag{2}$$

Table 4 summarises the results obtained when using the nine models.

Table 4. Classifiers Performances.

Classifiers	Best performance			
	%Accuracy (avg.)	%Accuracy	%Recall (class 0)	%Recall (class 1)
Decision tree	61.3	78.0	83.0	69.0
SVM	65.0	65.0	92.0	25.0
kNN	68.0	68.0	92.0	31.0
Boosted Tree	78.0	78.0	75.0	81.0
Bagged Tree	70.0	70.0	71.0	69.0
Subspace kNN	69.9	80.0	83.0	75.0
Subspace Discriminant	66.0	78.0	88.0	62.0
Majority vote 1	71.9	82.0	83.0	81.0
Majority vote 2	76.9	**85.0**	**88.0**	**81.0**

5   Discussion

The difference between the two genders is an important factor in determining human health. The medical knowledge about gender differences in anatomy, physiology, genetics support prognostic and diagnostic of diseases, e.g., cardiovascular diseases present different risk factors for men and women.

The gender identification using ECG signals can be useful in home-care systems, remote screening device for pathological rhythms or as ECG-based biometric system.

The 12-lead ECG configuration presents several advantages in terms of signal quality and interpretability, but nonstandard ECGs configurations allow data collection outside of a clinical context.

In this study, gender classification was conducted using nonstandard ECGs, resorting to CYBHi and ALLab datasets. CYBHi dataset comprises short-term and long-term signals, we used both signals to train our models. Allab dataset comprises short-term signals, and it was used for evaluating the models. The experimental settings of these two datasets were different, but the signals were collected with the same sampling rate (1000 Hz). The differences in experimental settings can compromise the good classification of genders, but nowadays it is possible to collect ECG using wearable devices in chest, wrist, or hands. We are aware that the orientation of the leads affects the morphology and amplitude of the measured ECG but in other side increase usability and allow more versatile solutions.

Another concern we had was to present a real and balanced training dataset without resorting to synthetic data.

Different classifiers are implemented, the results presented in Table 4 show that the better models are Boosted tree, Bagged tree and Subspace kNN with average accuracy from 78.0%; 70.0% and 69.9%. How we can verify the difference in the results is related to the behavior of each classifier, so, we also proposed resort to the majority vote to obtain two consensus decisions: 1. Boosted tree and Subspace kNN and 2. Boosted tree, Bagged tree and Subspace kNN. Both achieved a better recall balance.

The heart changes as we get older, and this is reflected in the features visible on the ECG. As a result, we may conclude that the difference in class results is directly influenced by this component [18].

These consensus decision results suggest the importance of feature selection. Table 5 shows the more important features for the method based on the majority vote using Boosted Tree, Bagged tree and Susbspace kNN. Generally, RR interval (mean and variability), duration of QRS (mean, variability, maximum), amplitude of QRS (mean, variability, maximum and minimum), QT interval (variability, maximum and minimum) and mean HR are the most important features.

Table 5. Feature importance.

Features	Models		
	Boosted Tree	Bagged tree	Subspace k-NN
mean RR		X	
Mean duration QRS	X		
Mean amplitude QRS	X		X
QT variability			X
RR variability	X		
QRS duration variability		X	
QRS amplitude variability			X
Maximum QT		X	
Minimum QT	X		
Maximum QRS duration	X		
Maximum QRS amplitude			X
Minimum QRS amplitude	X		
Mean HR		X	X

Automatic gender identification was tried by Tripathy et al. [13], Ergin et al. [9], Lyle et al. [17], Cabra et al. [7], Attia et al. [4], Goshvarpour & Goshvarpour [10], Khan et al. [12], and Al Alkeem et al. [1] with results above 90%. However, we tried and only got 85.0. We think that the previous papers may have had better results because length of the test dataset [9,13], unbalanced datasets [9], additional features [10,17], synthetic data [1,7] or data augmentation [1], noise addition [1] and internal validation [4,10,12].

In our view, what is needed is the proposal of a versatile framework for gender identification that allows realistic classifications. Our current approach uses real ECG signals to train the models and external validation. Besides, the ECG signals are collected using nonstandard configuration and settings, allowing usability in different context. So, in future work, we intend to propose a framework that can be incorporated as a gender identification module.

6   Conclusion

Many cardiovascular diseases (CVD) have more prevalence in women than men (angina pectoris, stroke) and inversely (coronary heart disease "CHD", heart failure), so the automatic detection of gender by ECG could be very important and improve the development of predictive systems for CVD and also in mobile or remote healthcare.

Considering the type of used ECG signals which can be collected from IoT devices, the proposed method can have several applications such as: reducing the data in face recognition research; improving CVD and other diseases with computer-aied diagnosis. in telemonitoring of where patient information is limited or in a monitoring center with cross information.

The main findings of this work are summarised as follows:

- Our method offers a realistic gender classification based on a simple feature extraction using nonstandard ECG signal;
- Bossted tree model provides good balance between each gender classification using a balanced dataset to train;
- The results from Bossted tree, Bagged tree and Subspace kNN suggest that feature selection improve the classification;
- A consensus decision can be used to improve and balance the classifications.

This work presents some limitations as a small dataset to train the models and the non-distinction between patients age, which can vary HRV features and QRS amplitude. So, in future work we are considering use ECG-ID dataset to apply our framework and added a new module for analysis of age similarities.

References

1. Alkeem, E.A., et al.: Robust deep identification using ECG and multimodal biometrics for industrial internet of things. Ad Hoc Netw. **121**, 102581 (2021)
2. ALLab: Signals from the Susana experiment. https://allab.di.ubi.pt/mediawiki/index.php/June_2017_Signals_from_the_Susana_experiment
3. Ashour, A.S., Guo, Y., Hawas, A.R., Xu, G.: Ensemble of subspace discriminant classifiers for schistosomal liver fibrosis staging in mice microscopic images. Health Inf. Sci. Syst. **6**(1), 1–10 (2018)

4. Attia, Z.I., et al.: Age and sex estimation using artificial intelligence from standard 12-lead ECGs. Circul. Arrhythmia Electrophysiol. **12**(9), 1–11 (2019). https://doi.org/10.1161/CIRCEP.119.007284
5. Awal, M., Mostafa, S., Ahmad, M.: Performance analysis of savitzky-golay smoothing filter using ecg signal. Int. J. Comput. Inf. Technol. **1**, 24 (2011)
6. Bansal, A., Joshi, R.: Portable out-of-hospital electrocardiography: a review of current technologies. J. Arrhythmia **34**(2), 129–138 (2018). https://doi.org/10.1002/joa3.12035
7. Cabra, J.L., Mendez, D., Trujillo, L.C.: Wide machine learning algorithms evaluation applied to ECG authentication and gender recognition. In: ACM International Conference Proceeding Series, pp. 6–12 (2018). https://doi.org/10.1145/3230820.3230830
8. Karius, D.R.: ECG primer: calculations. https://courses.kcumb.edu/physio/ecgprimer/normecgcalcs.htm
9. Ergin, S., Uysal, A.K., Gunal, E.S., Gunal, S., Gulmezoglu, M.B.: ECG based biometric authentication using ensemble of features. In: Iberian Conference on Information Systems and Technologies, CISTI (2014). https://doi.org/10.1109/CISTI.2014.6877089
10. Goshvarpour, A., Goshvarpour, A.: Gender and age classification using a new Poincare section-based feature set of ECG. Signal Image Video Process. **13**(3), 531–539 (2019)
11. Hargittai, S.: Savitzky-golay least-squares polynomial filters in ECG signal processing. Comput. Cardiol. **2005**, 763–766 (2005). https://doi.org/10.1109/CIC.2005.1588216
12. Khan, M.U., Saad, M., Aziz, S., Mumtaz, C.J., Naqvi, S.Z.H., Qasim, M.A.: Electrocardiogram based Gender Classification. In: 2nd International Conference on Electrical, Communication and Computer Engineering, ICECCE 2020, pp. 12–13 (2020). https://doi.org/10.1109/ICECCE49384.2020.9179305
13. Tripathy, R.K., Acharya, A., Choudhary, S.K.: Gender classification from ECG signal analysis using least square support vector machine. Am. J. Sig. Process. **2**(5), 145–149 (2012). https://doi.org/10.5923/j.ajsp.20120205.08
14. Kumar, N., Saini, D., Froelicher, V.: A gender-based analysis of high school athletes using computerized electrocardiogram measurements. PLoS ONE **8**(1), e53365 (2013). https://doi.org/10.1371/journal.pone.0053365
15. Li, Y., Zhang, S., Snyder, M.P., Meador, K.J.: Precision medicine in women with epilepsy: the challenge, systematic review, and future direction (2021). https://doi.org/10.1016/j.yebeh.2021.107928
16. Lin, F., Wu, Y., Zhuang, Y., Long, X., Xu, W.: Human gender classification: a review (2016). https://doi.org/10.1504/IJBM.2016.082604
17. Lyle, J.V., et al.: Beyond HRV: analysis of ECG signals using attractor reconstruction. Comput. Cardiol. **44**, 1–4 (2017). https://doi.org/10.22489/CinC.2017.091-096
18. Macfarlane, P.W.: The influence of age and sex on the electrocardiogram. Adv. Exp. Med. Biol. **1065**, 93–106 (2018). https://doi.org/10.1007/978-3-319-77932-4_6
19. Machluf, Y., Chaiter, Y., Tal, O.: Gender medicine: lessons from COVID-19 and other medical conditions for designing health policy. World J. Clin. Cases **8**(17), 3645–3668 (2020). https://doi.org/10.12998/wjcc.v8.i17.3645
20. Mauvais-Jarvis, F., et al.: Sex and gender: modifiers of health, disease, and medicine. Lancet **396**(January), 565–582 (2020)

21. orrite, C., Rodriguez, M., Martínez-Contreras, F., Fairhurst, M.: Classifier ensemble generation for the majority vote rule, vol. 5197, pp. 340–347 (2008). https://doi.org/10.1007/978-3-540-85920-8_42
22. Pedregosa, F., et al.: Scikit-learn: Machine learning in python. J. Mach. Learn. Res. **12**, 2825–2830 (2011)
23. Plaia, A., Buscemi, S., Fürnkranz, J., Mencía, E.L.: Comparing boosting and bagging for decision trees of rankings. J. Classification **39**(1), 78–99 (2022)
24. Plux, W.B.: Open signals. https://bitalino.com/en/software
25. Rajakariar, K., Koshy, A.N., Sajeev, J.K., Nair, S., Roberts, L., Teh, A.W.: Accuracy of a smartwatch based single-lead electrocardiogram device in detection of atrial fibrillation. Heart **106**(9), 665–670 (2020). https://doi.org/10.1136/heartjnl-2019-316004
26. Reale, C., Invernizzi, F., Panteghini, C., Garavaglia, B.: Genetics, sex, and gender (2021). https://doi.org/10.1002/jnr.24945
27. Regitz-Zagrosek, V.: Sex and gender differences in health. Sci. Soc. Ser. Sex Sci. EMBO Rep. **13**(7), 596–603 (2012). https://doi.org/10.1038/embor.2012.87
28. Romiti, G.F., Recchia, F., Zito, A., Visioli, G., Basili, S., Raparelli, V.: Sex and gender-related issues in heart failure (2020). https://doi.org/10.1016/j.hfc.2019.08.005
29. Safavian, S., Landgrebe, D.: A survey of decision tree classifier methodology. IEEE Trans. Syst. Man Cybern. **21**(3), 660–674 (1991). https://doi.org/10.1109/21.97458
30. Savitzky, A., Golay, M.J.E.: Smoothing and differentiation of data by simplified least squares procedures. Anal. Chemis. **36**(8), 1627–1639 (1964). https://doi.org/10.1021/ac60214a047
31. Sciences: school of health sciences - cardiology teaching package. https://www.nottingham.ac.uk/nursing/practice/resources/cardiology/function/normal_duration.php
32. da Silva, H.P., Lourenço, A., Fred, A., Raposo, N., Aires-de Sousa, M.: Check your biosignals here: a new dataset for off-the-person ECG biometrics. Comput. Methods Programs Biomed. **113**(2), 503–514 (2014). https://doi.org/10.1016/j.cmpb.2013.11.017
33. Xu, W., Zhuang, Y., Long, X., Wu, Y., Lin, F.: Human gender classification: a review. Int. J. Biometr. **8**, 275 (2016). https://doi.org/10.1504/IJBM.2016.10003589
34. Xue, J., Farrell, R.M.: How can computerized interpretation algorithms adapt to gender/age differences in ECG measurements. J. Electrocardiol. **47**(6), 849–855 (2014)
35. Yang, Y., Li, J., Yang, Y.: The research of the fast SVM classifier method. In: 2015 12th International Computer Conference on Wavelet Active Media Technology and Information Processing (ICCWAMTIP), pp. 121–124 (2015). https://doi.org/10.1109/ICCWAMTIP.2015.7493959

Designing a Soft-Actuated Smart Garment for Postural Control and Fall Prevention in Elderly Women

Alessia Buffagni(✉)

Università Iuav di Venezia, Santa Croce 191, 30135 Venezia, Italy
abuffagni@iuav.it

Abstract. A fall in third age triggers a domino effect of consequences that are recognized by specialists as leading causes of further falls. After the first event, the post-fall syndrome onsets: a pathological fear of falling that affects quality of life. It leads to loss of self-efficacy, sedentarism, musculoskeletal weakening, reduced mobility, postural insufficiency, gait disorders, isolation and depression—all acknowledged as fall risk factors. Specialists agreed that the most effective approach to prevent new episodes is to restore confident postures and good alignments. This paper presents the first design stages of a soft-actuated re-educational garment for remote post-fall rehabilitation in female users. The objective is to i) restore postural control by providing a gentle pressure stimulus, suggesting corrections when poor body alignments are detected; ii) restore the perceived self-efficacy; iii) promote physical activity by motion monitoring and providing daily reports through a patient-therapist smartphone app. To date, we have tested a soft body-postures detection system by cross-checking data from a network of e-textile stretch sensors, along with a pneumatic actuator system around the user's torso providing a targeted pressure stimulus to correct bad habits. Tests have been run on a limited number of users due to the Covid-19 emergency. Data are not yet statistically conclusive but suggest the way to a new dimensional approach, both for rehabilitation and prevention.

Keywords: Smart clothing · Remote rehabilitation · Post-fall syndrome

1 Introduction

One of the main causes of falling among seniors is having already fallen [1]. A fall in third age triggers physical, psychological, and social decline, which is most of the time irreversible [2]. After the first event, a disabling syndrome onsets. They call it the post-fall syndrome [3]. The elderly develop a pathological fear of falling again whose primary symptom is a progressive postural insufficiency [4, 5]. It, in turn, triggers a domino effect of consequences: loss of self-efficacy, sedentarism, weakening of musculoskeletal system, reduced mobility, isolation, and depression—all consistent risk factors for further falls [3]. This is why researchers and specialists agree that, when dealing with fear,

S. Spinsante et al. (Eds.): HealthyIoT 2022, LNICST 456, pp. 121–135, 2023.
https://doi.org/10.1007/978-3-031-28663-6_10

cognitive-behavioral interventions are highly advisable [6]. To date, the design science does not seem to have devoted much interest toward this disabling syndrome. Therefore, the question arises: is there a technology, or a combination of them, that might mitigate, and perhaps reverse, this functional decline? Systems for fall detection and prevention have been under examination for decades [7, 8]. Scientific research engines, such as Google Scholar or PubMed, provide a considerable amount of studies. However, by limiting the search to wearables, we can notice that little attention has been paid on smart garments as possible resources to develop and invest in. This study tries to somewhat remedy this shortcoming.

Designing a smart garment that 'senses' and anticipates the precise moment when the risk of falling may cause an injury is a challenge. Instead, to clothe seniors with something that might re-educate them and raise their awareness to the risk, stimulating their intrinsic abilities and perceived self-efficacy [9] is a goal that specialists recognize as worthy and valuable for practical verification. They agree that the most effective approach to prevent new episodes is to reinstate safe and confident posture and proper body alignment: regaining postural control is the essential condition for physical and psychological recovery. The end point of the patient's journey, regardless of the outcome of the first fall episode, is always a postural and gait retraining that prevents recurrences [10]. This research aims to design a soft-actuated re-educational garment for post-fall rehabilitation in female users—in every cultural and geographic context, women are the most affected individuals [11]: they outnumber men by 40–60% in terms of injury rate, and by 81% in terms of hospitalization rate [12]. This wearable system has the objective to i) restore postural control, muscular strength and balance, by providing a gentle pressure stimulus, suggesting corrections when poor body alignments are detected; ii) restore the perceived self-efficacy relying on the 'enclothed cognition' factor, according to which the design and functions of the garment influence the wearers' psychological and decision-making processes [13]; iii) promote physical activity by motion monitoring and providing daily reports through a patient-therapist smartphone application.

To date, we have tested a soft body-postures detection system by cross-checking data from a network of e-textile stretch sensors, along with a pneumatic actuator system around the user's torso (qualitative test) conceived to provide targeted pressure stimuli. The first version of the garment is a full-body suit (shirt, waistband, and pant-legs) designed to smoothly integrate these technologies into three fabric layers: second skin, e-textile, and outer layer. The soft actuation and posture detection would be driven by the fourth (intelligent) layer: a soft lumbar device that, besides housing electronics and mechanics, serves as a cushion to maintain correct posture while sitting (see Fig. 1). This device will collect and process data and will be connected to a patient-therapist smartphone application—not detailed in this paper.

2   Method

2.1   Soft Posture Detection

To detect body posture and alignment, we selected the technology that best fits fabrics without stiffness and bulges and with the least impact on manufacturing processes [14]: the *Machine-stitched E-textile Stretch Sensor* a conductive thread weaved onto stretchable fabric using the *bottom cover-stitch* technique. This is a loop pattern whose elongation leads to a drop in the electrical resistance measured at the sensor ends (see Fig. 2 and its caption).

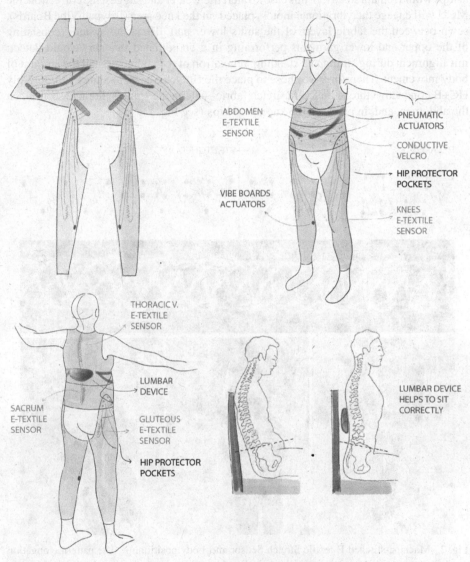

Fig. 1. Full-body smart suit scheme.

As previously investigated by Gioberto, Compton and Dunne [14], by attaching it to body areas in flexion and extension, body motion and position can be recognized and quantified. The Micro Controller Unit (MCU) provided for the operation of the system will read the data and activate the soft actuation. In such a simple way, the system can detect walking (alternating knee data detections) and sitting/standing position (simultaneous knee data detections). In addition, by placing a pair of sensors in the hip area, the system can recognize prolonged knee flexions and wrong weight unloading while standing: electrical resistance on knees' sensors would decrease while resistance at hips would remain steady. In this case, to alert the wearer and suggest the correction, the MCU will engage the vibrational motors placed on the knee area (Lilypad Vibe Boards), sewn between the fabric layers of the suit's lower part. Thus, the system (consisting of the upper and lower garments performing in a coordinated manner) would detect: misalignment during sitting and standing; relaxation of the abdomen; and the amount of body movement. Therefore, we chose to place the Stretch Sensor—Statex 235/36 2-ply HC+B conductive thread on Lycra stretch fabric—along the spine's thoracic section, on the abdomen, and, in pairs, on the knees and hips (see Fig. 2).

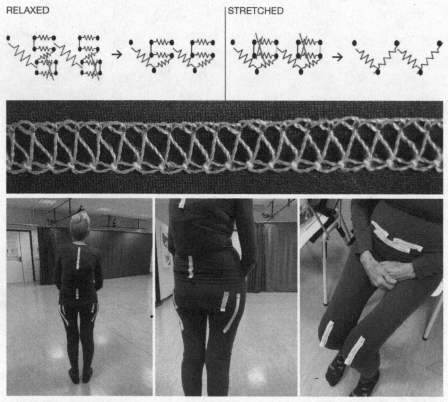

Fig. 2. Machine-stitched E-textile Stretch Sensor and body positioning. The pattern elongation causes a progression of contacts which gradually shorten the circuit, i.e. the electrical resistance measured at its ends. The longer the string (and the loop pattern recurrence), the more short-circuits induced by its elongation—and more effective the detection. For accurate details please refer to Gioberto, Compton and Dunne's study [14].

2.2 Soft Actuation

As abovementioned, when the MCU detects improper bending and trunk anteflexion a pneumatic soft actuator will be activated providing the corrective stimuli to the wearer, that must be perceptible for a certain amount of time. In order to prevent monotony, which is the enemy of receptivity, they should vary in intensity. We assigned this function to shape-transition pneumatic actuators (to be sewed inside the shirt), so that the air injection compresses the targeted body area and induces variable tones of stimulation. The alerting/stimulating engagement would vary as needed: *gentle*, at first, as a soft warning; *deeper*, as further warning; *intense*, when the wearer persists in improper posture.

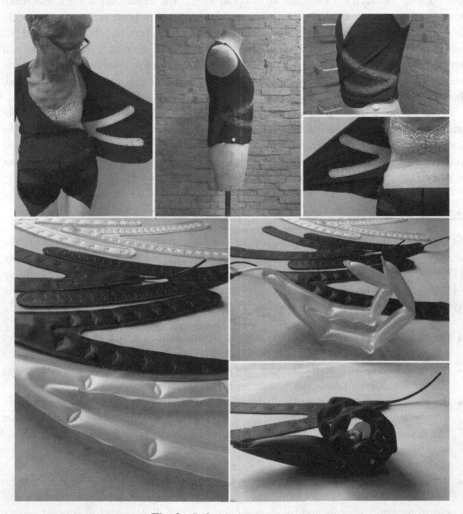

Fig. 3. Soft actuators prototypes.

Along with specialists of San Marco Rehabilitation Centre of Vicenza (Italy), we decided to place a pair of Y-shaped actuators on the abdomen area, between the chest and the lower abdomen. As tested, the stimulus would generate a more instinctive (hence, natural) corrective reaction—in addition, haptic perception and proprioceptive effect would be more intense. The structure and material of these actuators are crucial. The model we refer to is the *aeroMorph* [16], an advance study on origami patterns design for shape transition materials through air injection. As tested, by heat-printing strings of pre-tested geometric shapes onto one side of the actuator, it is possible to control bending during air injection.

Test-actuators have been prototyped in two versions (see Fig. 3): a lighter one, made of two layers of white TPU; and a stronger one, made of black TPU and a Cordura-coated side—to verify if a thicker layer could deflect the expansion inward, and make the stimulus more perceptible on the targeted body area. For each version, two models have been developed: a *six heat-printed diamonds* model, from which a segmented but yet fluid bending was expected; and a *sixteen heat-printed diamonds* one, to result in a spiral bending. The goal is to deliver a stimulating and yet not uncomfortable kinetic response, so it is crucial to avoid pumping air at pressures that require high-powered, bulky pumps.

The *six* and *sixteen diamonds* samples reacted to the air injection in a more suitable manner for the desired function, and with deformations compatible with the fabric and cut of the garment to be fixed into. We tested them along with the stretchable fabric and the human body (the shapes of which, especially if in the presence of adipose tissue, could mitigate, if not neutralize, the stimulus to be induced).

2.3   Garment Design

In order to find the proper balance between fabrics and components (acceptable to the wearer) we opted for the *layering system*, as recommended by Timmins and McCann [17]. The tailoring of both the upper and lower part of the system requires the assembling of three textile layers. A fourth 'layer' (not strictly textile) will be connected to the whole system through the upper part. Therefore, we designed:

- the intimate layer ('second skin') made of bi-elastic cotton (90% cotton, 10% elastane) which is soft, warm and gentle to the skin;
- the middle layer ('e-textile') made of Lycra where the sensor circuits are sewed (function accuracy takes priority over softness);
- the outer layer ('actuator-aesthetic') made of colored Lycra, where actuators adhere to its inner side—pneumatic ones in the upper garment and vibe boards in in the lower one (the outer side, essentially aesthetic, is provided with a *soft socket* in the lumbar area of the shirt to allow connection to the fourth 'layer', and side-pant pockets for optional hip protectors housing);
- the intelligent layer (not strictly a textile layer), a *plug-and-play* lumbar device to be attached to the soft socket of the upper garment (see Fig. 4). It hosts mechanics and electronics and is protected by an ergonomic soft shell designed to support proper sitting. Internally, there will be eight primary components at work: i) a MCU: for the first version of the system, we opted for SparkFun ESP32 Thing board which integrates

ii) a Bluetooth module; iii) an air micro-pump (diameter: 27 mm; length: 60 mm; weight: 60 g, noise: <55 db; voltage: 6.0 V; emission: 2 l/min); iv) a 3.7 V (7.4 W, 2000 mAh) battery pair in series; v) a solenoid valve; vi) a pressure sensor and vii) additional Printed Circuit Boards (PCB) for transistors and microresistors placement (required for sensor signals readability); and viii) a USB input for recharging.

The suit's full-version is designed as a modular combination: wrap shirt, lumbar device, waistband, and pant-legs—whose design is not detailed in this paper. Cuts and shapes are the result of multiple wearability tests on elder female users in attempt to find the best mediation between wearability, usability, acceptability and garment performance.

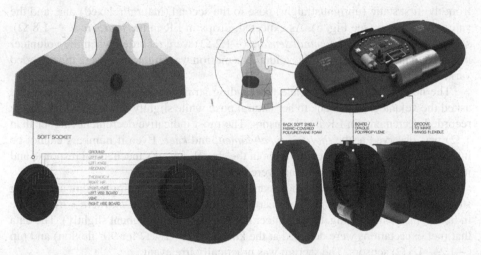

Fig. 4. The 'intelligent layer'(socket and lumbar device).

3 Results

3.1 Experimental Analysis

To run the experimental analysis, we used a standard stretchable suit functional for keeping sensors exposed and easily reachable by digital multimeter probes. The tested volunteer was 75 year old woman with thoracic hyperkyphosis, asymmetrical shoulders, and protracted abdomen. As agreed with physiatrists, we tested:

- One thoracic vertebral sensor: 15 cm, vertical, along the thoracic section of the spine—from T1 to T8 vertebrae—to detect back slouching;
- One sacral sensor: 10 cm, vertical, along the sacral section—from L4 to Sacrum—to support /confirm data from the thoracic vertebral sensor;
- One abdomen sensor: 15 cm, below the navel, horizontal, to detect abdominal relaxation;

- Two hip sensors: 15 cm, vertical, between the gluteus maximus muscle and the biceps femoris longus muscle, to detect sitting, standing, and motion along with the knee sensors.
- Two knee sensors: 5 cm, vertical, between the quadriceps femoris tendon and the patella, to detect sitting, standing, motion, and incorrect weight unloading along with the hip sensors.

 The technical protocol combines the employment of the digital multimeter with postures and steps analysis processed by a Vicon optoelectrical motion capture system— to verify the effective extent of movement that produced the Electrical Resistance (ER) variation. Data obtained from two sets of static poses and one moderate pace walk have been cross-referenced. Tables 1, 2 and 3 show the ER of each stretch sensor in transition from the first static (upright/straight) pose to the second (natural/relaxed) one, and the value of variation (see Fig. 5). As expected, drops in ER in the *thoracic v.* ($-1.8\ \Omega$), *sacrum* ($-0.6\ \Omega$), and *abdominal sensors* ($-1.2\ \Omega$) were recorded when the volunteer indulged in incorrect posture. The volunteer's motion was slight, so as were the recorded variations.

 The next static detections relate to: standing straight toward standing relaxed (we asked the volunteer to go back to her natural pose while slightly flexing her knees). We recorded decrements in ER in all sensors. The most indicative decrement (higher than $1\ \Omega$) was observed at the *thoracic v.*, *abdomen*, and *knee*. Even if numbers cannot be intended as conclusive, expectations about the stretch sensor's mechanical response and its reliability in most body segments were met [18].

 As a completion of the static poses analysis, we crossed standing upright and sitting straight. As expected, most values decreased (the small rise in *thoracic v.* resistance indicates that, while sitting, the volunteer improved spinal alignment slightly). The data that met expectations were detected at the knee ($-2.6/-2.4\ \Omega$ for 90° flexion) and hip ($-4.2/-4.3\ \Omega$) sensors. The sacrum was practically irrelevant.

Table 1. Static posture detection: sitting.

Sensor	Sitting upright	Sitting relaxed	ER variation
Thoracic V	$56,2\ \Omega$	$54,4\ \Omega$	$-1,8\ \Omega$
Sacrum	$27,5\ \Omega$	$26,9\ \Omega$	$-0,6\ \Omega$
Abdomen	$28,3\ \Omega$	$27,1\ \Omega$	$-1,2\ \Omega$
L HIP	$46,1\ \Omega$	$46,1\ \Omega$	–
R Hip	$45,6\ \Omega$	$45,6\ \Omega$	–
L Knee	$17,6\ \Omega$	$18,1\ \Omega$	$+0,5\ \Omega$
R Knee	$17,2\ \Omega$	$17,8\ \Omega$	$+0,6\ \Omega$

 The legs' sensor-equipment also serves as a soft motion recording instrument, allowing to monitor the degree of activity or sedentarism of the wearer without overloading the MCU with additional data from Inertial Measurement Unit (IMU) sensors. Thus, we also

Table 2. Static posture detection: standing.

Sensor	Standing straight	Standing naturally (flexed knees)	ER Variation
Thoracic V	55,8 Ω	54,4 Ω	−1,4 Ω
Sacrum	28,0 Ω	27,9 Ω	−0,1 Ω
Abdomen	28,9 Ω	27,2 Ω	−1,7 Ω
L Hip	50,3 Ω	50,2 Ω	−0,1 Ω
R Hip	49,9 Ω	49,7 Ω	−0,2 Ω
L Knee	20,2 Ω	18,8 Ω	−1,4 Ω
R Knee	19,6 Ω	18,5 Ω	−1,1 Ω

Table 3. Static posture detection: standing vs sitting.

Sensor	Standing straight	Sitting upright	ER variation
Thoracic V	55,8 Ω	56,2 Ω	+0,4 Ω
Sacrum	28,0 Ω	27,5 Ω	−0,5 Ω
Abdomen	28,9 Ω	28,3 Ω	−0,6 Ω
L Hip	50,3 Ω	46,1 Ω	−4,2 Ω
R Hip	49,9 Ω	45,6 Ω	−4,3 Ω
L Knee	20,2 Ω	17,6 Ω	−2,6 Ω
R Knee	19,6 Ω	17,2 Ω	−2,4 Ω

tested the sensor's accuracy for this function (Table 4, see Fig. 6). First, we examined the *hip* sensor. While static, the measured ER was 36 Ω. While walking, it went from 34.2 Ω (min) to 38.6 Ω (max). Peaks relate to maximum flexor traction (initial swing phase), and relaxation (terminal swing phase). The ER variation (4.4 Ω) met expectations [18]. The recurrence of such a value variation will enable the MCU to detect and quantify the motion while wearing the system. Similarly, the *knee* sensor was tested. While walking, the resistance oscillated from 18.3 to 20.4 Ω. (19.2 at rest). This variation (2.1 Ω) was sufficient for the purpose.

At the conclusion of the session, it can be assumed that, by cross-referencing the data detected by the e-textile stretch sensors, the intelligent layer will be able to distinguish right from wrong postures, and walking from sitting [18].

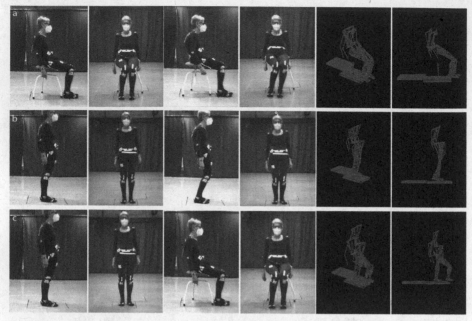

Fig. 5. a) sitting upright and relaxed compared; b) standing straight and naturally (with flexed knees) compared; c) standing straight and sitting upright compared.

Table 4. Walking detection.

Sensor	Static	Swing (max flexion)	Stance (max extension)	ER Variation
R Hip	36,0 Ω	34,2 Ω	38,6 Ω	4,4 Ω
R Knee	19,2 Ω	18,3 Ω	20,4 Ω	2,1 Ω

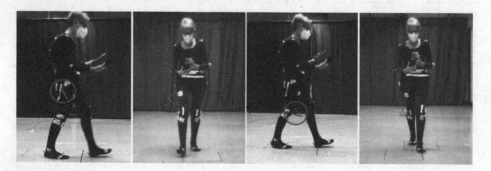

Fig. 6. Walking detection.

3.2   The Pneumatic Actuators: Qualitative Experimental Analysis of the Tactile-Compressive Function

Qualitative experimental analysis was based on subjective reports. While we were able to assess the proper actuators' kinetic response to the transit of air, we could not rely on objective protocols to measure a patient's sensation [18]. Our m. o. had to be sympathetic, i.e. the attentive listen to the volunteers and their physical and mental involvement through the experimentation. Tests were carried out in two phases: the first one with three volunteers—we tested different combination of actuators to verify which version and pattern is more perceptible—and the second one, with two patients in postural rehabilitation (social restriction imposed by the 2020/21 pandemic emergency has made contact with vulnerable people limited) by integrating the chosen actuators into the mock-up shirt as described in Sect. 2.3 *Garment design*.

The first volunteer (v.1), aged 75 years, suffered from previous fall episodes, she has gynoid body conformation and adipose tissue in the contact areas of the actuators (see Fig. 7).

Test 1: during both standing and sitting, v.1 put on the six diamond samples in pairs between two Lycra shirts—first the light version, then the reinforced one (see Fig. 7). She was asked to indicate the points where the given stimulus was most pronounced when we injected air and to refer her sensation. She reported that with both versions there is a clear sensation of pressure is perceptible, and spread around the belly. Nonetheless, the white one [light] displayed a more peculiar touch.

Test 2: v.1 was asked to try both versions with sixteen diamonds, and again indicate which spots were most stimulated. She reported she felt an air flow very similar to the previous test, but this time there was a kind of slightly stronger manipulation, especially with the black version [Cordura-coated], under the chest and the navel [i.e., at the extremities of the actuator, where the shrinkage is most detectable—especially in the reinforced samples]. While in doubt about which density was preferable (light or strong), v.1 preferred the sixteen-diamond model for each version. V.1 reported three substantial factors: i) a preferable *fit to the body* was perceived (whereas the six-diamond samples provided the sensation of detaching from the torso as the volume increased); ii) a vigorous *manipulation* was perceived in the central abdominal area; iii) on a merely aesthetic perspective, the pattern emerging from the fabric looked more graceful than the *sausage pattern* generated by the six-diamond sample—the defect was visible in both versions, implying that the Cordura coating did not drive the deformation inward as effectively as expected.

The session was repeated three days later to let receptors' memories vanish. This time we tested the light and Cordura-coated versions of each sample in combination. We repeated test 1 and 2 twice. The second time we gave v.1 the handpump so that she could take control of the air injection and ponder the sensory involvement by herself in proportion to the pressure and volume of the pumped fluid. At the conclusion of the new session, uncertainty about materials persisted (after each new test, v.1 reported she *felt better* the lighter version). On the other side, impressions regarding the number of diamonds were strongly confirmed: lastly, v.1 reported that the folds of the sixteen-diamonds were more stimulating.

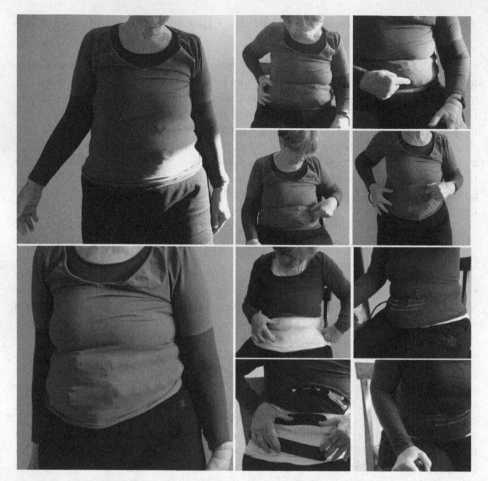

Fig. 7. First phase tests; untied samples test with volunteers.

We turned to volunteer 2 (v.2), aged 81 years old, who suffered from several previous fall episodes. She has android body conformation, taut belly without adipose mass. We proposed her the same sequence of tests. Her impressions were almost identical.

V.2 reported she felt more affected by the sample with sixteen diamonds and between black and white [light and reinforced] she didn't feel much difference. She felt the same pressure in the same spots. Eventually, she chose the white option because it made her feel less bulky, it is less rigid underneath the fabric, and it seemed to be less awkward.

The final volunteer (v.3), younger, aged 71, with one fall episode without injuries, android conformation, soft bellied but still toned, confirmed the same impressions.

Although leaving us hesitant about the usefulness of Cordura coating, tests on free samples (not yet sewn into the mock-up shirt) provided us unanimous confirmation: size, shape, and pattern withstand tests on different body conformations: the targeted body area—whether taut, soft with adipose mass, or relaxed—received the fluid stimulation with an intensity that met expectations.

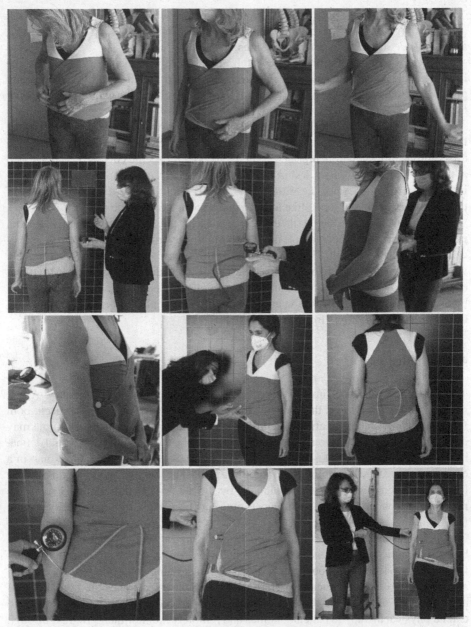

Fig. 8. Second phase tests; test of the mock-up with patients.

We then proceed with testing on patients at the rehabilitation centre (see Fig. 8). Thus, we basted the mock-up shirt, integrating the sixteen-diamond samples: the light version on the left side, and the reinforced one [Cordura-coated] on the right.

Patients undergoing postural rehabilitation therapy were 71 (p.1) and 64-year-old (p.2). The physiatrist started the sequence of tests by personally adjusting the air pressure, and asked p.1 and p.2 to report impressions.

As per P.1's report: the pressure was felt more strongly on the left [where there the lighter sample was]; the actuation, although *audible*, did not suggest how to correctly posture, even if, admittedly, a sort of *urge to react* was felt; on the end, the tightness of the garment was quite invigorating.

As per P.2's report: a more distinctive manipulation was detected on the left and middle side of the abdomen; the actuation was indeed pretty loud but did not keep the torso upright as it should [being accustomed to rigid orthopaedic corsets, P.2 envisioned a 'passive' administration, i.e. a shirt to keep her torso in an upright position without her intervention or effort]; once the shirt was taken off, it felt like there was still a *trace* of the actuation around the torso, like a *tactile memory* in that specific area.

Reports were consistent with expectations. The physiatrist explained that both patients were neither prepared nor, more importantly, instructed on how to react physically to the induced stimuli. They were brought into contact with the product deliberately without any previous mediation. This gave rise to their doubts about the 'active' re-educational function. If this smart garment is ever adopted as a therapeutic device, it will be up to the physician to prescribe and explain the proper physical response following the stimulus, which differs from case to case [18].

4 Conclusion

Tests have been run on a limited user sample due to the Covid-19 emergency. Albeit not statistically conclusive, they suggest the way to a new dimensional approach, both for rehabilitation and prevention. According to physiatrists, this assistive principle may indeed make sense: the neuromotor stimulus provided by the fluid injection would define, in the mid-term, an *intimate user-device language* that trains postural education—in a conscious way at the beginning until becoming almost irreflective, natural with practice [18]. Thus, the corrective reaction induced by the air flow would gradually reinforce muscles, consolidating better posture over time and, as a result, limiting the risk and the fear of falling.

In conclusion, the project's aims are several. First, it seeks to provide a comprehensive geriatric tool to physically and psychologically rehabilitate patients and prevent further falls. Second, to probe the effectiveness of a therapeutic pneumatic actuation as a tool for postural re-education. Third, to explore the effectiveness and durability of a new user-device dialogue through targeted stimulation on sensitive areas. Fourth, to extend physical therapy to patients' homes and remotely monitor their progress through a patient-therapist smartphone application—which has not been detailed in this paper. Fifth, to shorten recovery and reduce the risk of new falls—meaning, in turn, reducing direct and indirect costs, both for the individual and health systems.

Moreover, if ever needed, this paper also seeks to emphasize how a multidisciplinary approach, involving specialists, therapists, and end-users, is the key to design remote healthcare devices that are truly centred on user needs—and somewhat innovative compared to current tools and practices.

References

1. Young, W.R., Mark Williams, A.: How fear of falling can increase fall-risk in older adults: applying psychological theory to practical observations. Gait Posture **41**(1), 7–12 (2015)
2. Choi, K., Jeon, G.S., Cho, S.: Prospective study on the impact of fear of falling on functional decline among community dwelling elderly women. Int. J. Environ. Res. Public Health **14**(5), 1–11 (2017)
3. Lopes, K., Costa, D., Santos, L., Castro, D., Bastone, A.: Prevalence of fear of falling and its correlation. Rev. Bras. Fisioter. **13**(3), 223–229 (2009)
4. Kurz, I., Oddsson, L., Melzer, I.: Characteristics of balance control in older persons who fall with injury – a prospective study. J. Electromyogr. Kinesiol. **23**(4), 814–819 (2013)
5. Pfitzenmeyer, P., Mourey, F., Mischis-Troussard, C., Bonneval, P.: Rehabilitation of serious postural insufficiency after falling in very elderly subjects. Arch. Gerontol. Geriatr. **33**(3), 211–218 (2001)
6. Oude Voshaar, R.C., Banerjee, S., Horan, M., Baldwin, R., Pendleton, N., Proctor, R., et al.: Fear of falling more important than pain and depression for functional recovery after surgery for hip fracture in older people. Psychol. Med. **36**(11), 1635–1645 (2006)
7. Mubashir, M., Shao, L., Seed, L.: A survey on fall detection: principles and approaches. Neurocomputing **100**, 144–152 (2013)
8. Hamm, J., Money, A.G., Atwal, A., Paraskevopoulos, I.: Fall prevention intervention technologies: a conceptual framework and survey of the state of the art. J. Biomed. Inform. **59**, 319–345 (2016)
9. Bandura, A.: Self-Efficacy. The Corsini Encyclopedia of Psychology. Wiley, New York (2010)
10. Dionyssiotis, Y., Dontas, I.A., Economopoulos, D., Lyritis, G.P.: Rehabilitation after falls and fractures. J. Musculoskelet. Neuronal Interact. **8**(3), 244–250 (2008)
11. Rau, C.S., et al.: Geriatric hospitalizations in fall-related injuries. Scand. J. Trauma Resusc. Emerg. Med. **22**(1), 4–11 (2014)
12. Stevens, J.A., Sogolow, E.D.: Gender differences for non-fatal unintentional fall related injuries among older adults. Inj. Prev. **11**(2), 115–119 (2005)
13. Adam, H., Galinsky, A.D.: Enclothed cognition. J. Exp. Soc. Psychol. **48**(4), 918–925 (2012)
14. Gioberto, G., Compton, C., Dunne, L.E.: Machine-stitched e-textile stretch sensors. Sens. Transducers **202**(7), 25–37 (2016)
15. Perry, J.: Gait Analysis. Normal and pathological function. SLACK Incorporated, Thorofare (1992)
16. Ou, J., et al.: AeroMorph – heat-sealing inflatable shape-change materials for interaction design. In: UIST 2016 – Proceedings of the 29th Annual Symposium on User Interface Software and Technology, pp. 121–32 (2016)
17. Timmins, M.W., McCann, J.: Overview of the design requirements of the active ageing. In: McCann, J., Bryson, D. (eds.) Textile-led Design for the Active Ageing Population. Woodhead Publishing. Elsevier Ltd. (2015)
18. Buffagni, A.: Intelligent clothing for the ageing body. The pursuit of a design method. https://air.iuav.it/handle/11578/306340. Accessed 05 Sept 2022

Cultivate Smart and Healthy Ageing

Andreas Andreou[1]([✉]), Constandinos X. Mavromoustakis[1],
Evangelos Markakis[2], George Mastorakis[3], Jordi Mongay Batalla[4],
Evangelos Pallis[5], and Ciprian Dobre[6]

[1] Department of Computer Science, University of Nicosia and University of Nicosia
Research Foundation, Nicosia, Cyprus
{andreou.andreas,mavromoustakis.c}@unic.ac.cy
[2] Department of Electrical and Computer Engineering, Hellenic Mediterranean
University, Heraklion, Crete, Greece
markakis@pasiphae.eu
[3] Department of Management Science and Technology, Hellenic Mediterranean
University, Agios Nikolaos, Crete, Greece
gmastorakis@hmu.gr
[4] Warsaw University of Technology, Warsaw, Poland
jordi.mongay.batalla@pw.edu.pl
[5] Department of Industrial Design and Production Engineering,
School of Engineering, University of West Attica, Athens, Greece
epallis@uniwa.gr
[6] National Institute for Research and Development in Informatics,
Bucharest, Romania
ciprian.dobre@upb.ro

Abstract. The essential criterion for developing an intelligent age-friendly environment is evaluating and monitoring the provision of services. Our research aims to allow the deployment of a broad range of digital healthcare solutions interconnected in an IoT network ecosystem. Through their interoperability, we will be able to cultivate age-friendly smart homes for older adults. Thus, we will enable interpreted living and wellbeing. The intelligent integrations of digital solutions will allow the acquisition and evaluation of health-related data. Standardization, interoperability and scalability of the integration will increase efficiency in healthcare, improving older adults' Quality of Life (QoL). Also, interpreting their needs will allow key stakeholders to optimize the Quality of Service (QoS). The proposed Internet of Health (IoH) framework will encapsulate sustainable and affordable innovative solutions and their benefits for a comfortable, meaningful, and independent life in an intelligent environment. Therefore, the frame mediated by edge computing, in-home and community settings will be able to interact with healthcare networks contributing to hospitalizations and institutional care.

Keywords: Smart-Cities · Internet of Things · Age-Friendly · Internet of Health

S. Spinsante et al. (Eds.): HealthyIoT 2022, LNICST 456, pp. 136–147, 2023.
https://doi.org/10.1007/978-3-031-28663-6_11

1   Introduction

We propose developing a framework that will enable the development of a wide range of digital solutions and services to support and extend healthy and independent living for older adults. The framework will be made possible by integrating interoperable IoT platforms, which combine intelligent devices to acquire and evaluate data. The information will be about the vital signs, living environment and lifestyle of the elderly. Also, the information collected will determine their needs for independent living. Of utmost importance is ensuring data protection and trust, ensuring anonymity through personalized solutions. In addition, we focus on the interoperability and scalability of IoT networks to maintain remote efficiency in healthcare delivery, bringing well-being to seniors, supporting their families, empowering caregivers, and fostering innovation from care providers. The proposed framework will promote age-friendliness in home and community environments. Home accessibility will be assessed based on the WHO guidelines for housing and health for the elderly. They will also be able to evaluate the provision of services and identify possible psychosocial and physical modifications to enhance their independent living. We will also address age-friendliness in terms of attitudes and cultural values. Age-friendliness requires fostering attitudes and behaviours that promote older people's dignity and worth, a sense of safety, and being active members of society. The aim is to identify the views of older people on how to foster age-friendly behaviours, how the proposed framework can facilitate this and how people can be encouraged to use IoT solutions to promote recommendations for creating age-friendly. The main aim is to consider how older people and their carers should be engaged and empowered to play a more active role in healthcare decision-making to improve the overall quality of care, efficiency, and results. Ambitious but realistic goal setting can add a sense of purpose, drive, and achievement. In addition, they will be able to examine

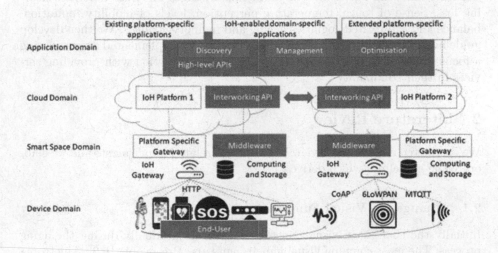

Fig. 1. Architecture of an IoH platform

how the psychology of decision-making and goal setting can be applied to facilitate older people's planning and guide development about the type and extent of information that is optimal to help older people to make decisions.

Healthcare platforms will intelligently enable semantic interoperability of the Internet of Health (IoH). The interconnection of digital healthcare solutions in an Internet of Things (IoT) network combined with services like Smart Home and Smart Mobility will enhance sustainability in Smart Cities and cultivate age-friendliness. Health-related data could be acquired remotely for evaluation. Thus, the users will have the opportunity of remote vital signs monitoring. However, to incentivize data sharing, we need to ensure that the exchange will be secure between trusted parties. Therefore, a middleware platform could support the secure exchange of data and services. Simple in terms of time complexity and robust in terms o secureness, novel cryptography methods could be deployed to assure data sovereignty [33,34]. As presented in Fig. 1 the IoH network ecosystem could perform in four domains. Within the application domain, the middleware platform will allow the integration of digital devices, healthcare services, and intelligent digital solutions [35]. The data will be accessible through the decryption key for interpretation through the cloud domain. Hence, it will provide consistent and valid access to virtualized IoH digital solutions. The intelligent space domain will deliver services for engaging innovative IoH devices in intelligent environments, allowing dynamic configuration of digital solutions. Finally, the device domain regards the devices that will consist of the IoH platform. The intelligent interaction with the innovative ecosystem of the smart urban environment will leverage their roaming capabilities [36].

First, we set out to conduct a systematic review of the literature on older adults experiencing permanently or temporarily reduced functionality and capabilities. Then, based on their disability, we provide the corresponding suggestions to promote digital solutions adapted to their needs. The areas we investigated were the following age-related impairments: Changes in visual function, Hearing loss, Sense of touch, temperature perception, levels of mobility limitation, balance and age-related cognitive ageing and memory changes. We then develop guidelines for presenting digital solutions. Finally, we implemented a survey using a focus group of 30 older people to assess their satisfaction with providing services in their community.

2   Literature Review

We conducted a literature review based on age-related impairments and we elaborate the guidelines which derives.

2.1   Changes in Visual Function

Initially the changes in visual function deteriorate gradually during the aging process. The most common visual impairments are: Presbyopia [1,2]; Ametropia [3,4]; Glare sensitivity; Cataract [5]; Dark adaptation [6–8]; A complex process mediates colour perception between neurons [9] and Tunnel vision [10–12]. The guidelines for visual presentation which derives from these changes are as follow: Raise illumination on reading surfaces; Use the matte screen surfaces; The need for stimuli should be large, simple, unobstructed, and in the central field of vision; Make things distinctive by increasing size (minimum font 12 points), using warm colors (avoid Violet, Blue, and Green) and by increasing contrast (50:1 contrast, e.g., LCD Screen) such as white text on black background [13]; Use fonts such as Arial, Helvetica, Times, Bookman, and Book Antigua without a script and decorative fonts distinctly; The uppercase letters attract attention but are not easy to read in long sections of text.

2.2   Decline in Hearing

The decline in hearing during aging cause the following auditory impairments: Presbycusis which is a common type of sensorineural decline of hearing through natural aging (i.e., Sound perception diminishes by 2.5 dB per decade up to age 55 and then accelerates to 8.5 dB per decade) [14]; Frequency discrimination performances deteriorate in an approximately linear manner with age (e.g., perception of high frequencies diminishes with age, especially in men) [15]; Different stimuli can cause sound localization disorientation in each ear due to age-related hearing loss and auditory selective attention affects performance in a multitasking environment and is the reason why it is difficult for seniors to process distinct sounds at a fast pace [16]. Based on barriers that we have already elaborated we conclude to the following guidelines for auditory presentation: An average conversational speech is about 50 dB due to that sound signals should be at least 60 db; The volume must be easy to adjust with simple gestures; Sound alerts should be within the frequency range of 500 to 2000 Hz, which is the standard speech range; It would be beneficial to avoid using synthesized or robotic speech patterns; It is necessary to signal an alert sound at a frequency higher than 2000 Hz we must use a longer duration (i.e., >0.5 s); To avoid high-frequency sounds, we can use cross-sensory channels such as vibration and flashing light [17]; Procurement of headphones will be an excellent solution to eliminate background sounds and disorientation and we need to maintain a high "signal-to-noise" ratio to eliminate reverberation.

2.3   Sense of Touch, the Perception of Temperature, Mobility Limitation Levels, and Balance

Aging has an impact on the sense of touch, the perception of temperature, mobility limitation levels, and balance. Therefore, we studied the most significant limitations which occur through aging process. Pressure sensitivity diminishes through aging, so it is harder to sense when the finger has made full contact with a surface or when a small feeling has been depressed [18]; Reduced thermal sensitivity because of limited nerve ending function and heat retention [19]; Reduced mobility capacity caused by loss of muscle strength, tone, and flexibility [20]; Balance impairment due to arthritics and tremor that occurs with aging cause diminished static postural control and diminished dynamic balance [21, 22]. We design guidelines for diminished temperature, touch sensation, movement restriction, and balance instability as follow: Avoid 3D touch screens; Use less complicated virtual devices [23]; Use supplemental sensory cues to warn of high temperatures; Prefer textured surfaces instead of smooth surfaces to complement the touch feel; A sound alert that a button on the screen or computer key has been depressed; Provide time for discrete movement tasks; Avoid multiple rapid steps (e.g., adjust double-click speed of computer mouse, tracking rate on scroll ball); Simple task movements for senior with tremor; Prefer levers than knobs; Large buttons rather than small ones; Use solid color carpets in case of sensor mat; Avoid unsecured objects (e.g., unsecured end-of-aisle displays present obstacles to motorized or static ambulatory aids.) in the case of robot assistant [24].

2.4   Cognitive Aging and Age-Related Changes in Memory

Short-term memory can be set to cache and manipulate stimuli no longer available to the senses. With aging, fewer discrete information bits processed at a given time, and information overload may occur [25]; Prospective memory refers to remembering to take a planned action in the future. Aging men can not jeopardize spontaneous recovery processes, but the ability to deactivate completed intentions is impaired [26]; Semantic memory refers to a long-term memory portion that processes ideas and general facts that do not come from personal experience. Semantic memory performance in the elderly reduces in processing speed and executive function [27]; Procedural memory defines as a type of long-term memory and unconscious memory of skills and how to act. Procedural memory usually does not decrease with age, but it takes longer for older people to learn new skills [28]; Age reduces attention, but the reduction does not include all components of attentive functioning equally [29]; Spatial cognition is a complex, multifaceted set of processes engaged in a large variety of tasks [30]. Spatial navigation is impairing after the age of 60, with acceleration in decline after 70 [31]; Language comprehension difficulties are interpreted as limitations on processing ability so that the requirements for simultaneous recording of superficial meaning and concurrent execution of integrative and constructive processes reduced with age [20]. The guidelines to accommodate age-related cognitive changes are as follow: Provide simple instructions into discrete short messages; Provide event reminders but without too many unnecessary gadgets; Procedures should be simple, intuitive steps with a slow pace and opportunities for practice; Avoid visual clutter or ambient noise and use simple screens with small dis-tinct signals; Avoid redundant information and use a predictable linguistic structure with clear messages reasonable pace; Use Natural Language Processing (NLP) toolkit [32]. Based on the literature review, we developed Table 1 which refers to the instructions for digital solution educators in older adults.

Table 1. Guidelines for Tutors of Digital Solution

Functional limitation	Guidelines for tutors of Digital Solution
Decline in hearing	Get the listener's attention before you speak
	Look at the listener as you speak
	Speak naturally
	Use simple words and sentence structure
	Avoid ambient noise
	Use visual signs and gestures
Cognitive impairment	Provide slow and clean lines of communication
	Use a calm and focused communication
	Be aware the listener may lack confidence
	Evaluate whether the listener understands
	Find another way to express the information
	if the listener does not seem to understand
Mobility limitations	Take a seat at the same level and apply eye contact with
	the listener/speaker
	Treat the potential wheelchair as part of the
	listener's/speaker's personal space
	Use natural lip movements, voice tone, and volume
	Use condescending language
	Use non-patronizing language and actions
Visual function impairments	Consult with the person as to the type of communication needed
	(e.g., large font, disk, Braille, text-to-speech)
	Use natural volume and tone
	Ask for feedback to evaluate if the listener understands
	Check related software and hardware for visually impaired people

3 Age-friendly, Integrated, Intergenerational Neighborhoods

The internet of things (IoT) has become inextricably linked with creating smart cities. As the name implies, smart cities are structured atop more intelligent data. It is a significant challenge because data is frequently an afterthought when it comes to creating new processes and opportunities. Using the right building blocks from the outset is vital, aligned with clear and compelling guidelines about best practices. To achieve scale, we need standards to qualify how we view and measure the world around us and how this data informs our decision-making processes. Figure 2 is designed to align participants around a clear shared goal and guide them to a common destination. Accelerate the construction of a new breed of age-friendly housing in 'smart' socially supportive multi-generational neighbourhoods, development of innovative technologies and service models to improve health and well-being to reduce the financial burden on citizens and the State based on the following aspects:

- Work: Opportunities to work; Provision of training; Work-life balance; Labour market participation;
- Access to healthcare: Distance; Waiting times; Affordability;
- Mental health: Sense of self-worth; Loneliness, isolation; Depression, anxiety; A sense of purpose; Sense of connectedness, belonging;
- Adult education: Information provision; IT literacy;
- Housing: Safe, secure; Connected; Age-friendly; Healthy;
- Services: Healthcare; Transport;
- Neighbourhood problems: Infrastructural issues; Sense of safety; Perception pf vulnerability; Anti-social behaviour;
- Social Support: Family and friends; Neighbours; Community organizations;
- Public Spaces: Pleasant, interesting; Safe; Accessible, close by; Enable self-determination; Foster activity.

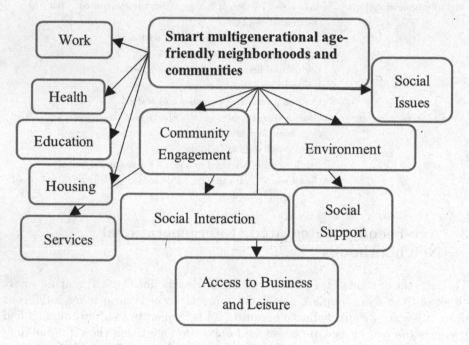

Fig. 2. Dependencies

4   Evaluation Results

We have implemented a survey among 30 older adults living in different districts of an urban environment through the Place Standard tool. We evaluated the provision of services by the community Fig. 3 and Fig. 4 show the responses obtained and plot them in two diagrams. The mean and median conclude with a look at the services performing well and where there is room for improvement. From the results, we conclude that all sections of service provision to the elderly need improvement.

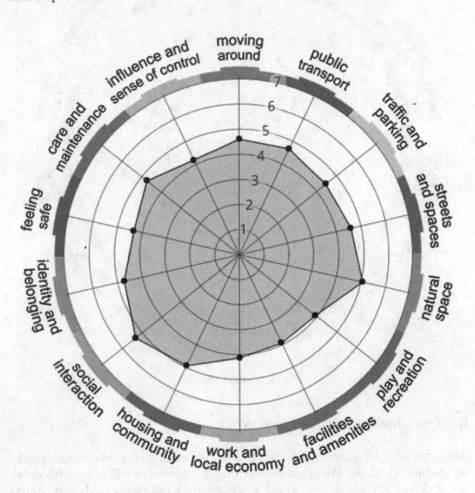

Fig. 3. Mean Results

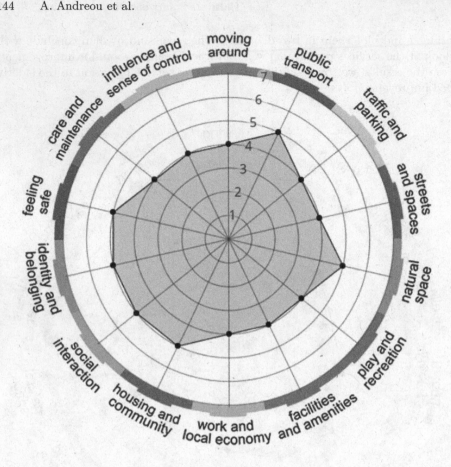

Fig. 4. Median Results

5   Conclusion and Future Work

Assessing age-friendliness in the city is a fundamental step in encouraging older adults' quality of life. We envisage that this research work will align with developing new standards for intelligent multi-generational neighbourhoods. Accessibility at home will be informed by the WHO Housing and Health guidelines, enabling older individuals to rate their private living space accessibility and identify possible psychosocial and physical modifications that will help sustain independent living. Therefore, age-friendliness necessitates cultivating attitudes and behaviours that promote the dignity and worth of older people, their sense of security and belonging, and being wanted and valued members of society. Ageing in place means more than continuing to live among the comforts and memories of home. Given the likelihood that we will live with the threat of pandemics for the foreseeable future, how might we pool resources to design age-friendly urban environments where public space doesn't become a no-go zone but remains a safe and habitable communal meeting point? Challenges lie at the heart of ongoing discussions with architects, designers, planners, social housing organizations, developers, health and social care service providers, technologists, local governments, researchers, and other AAA stakeholders. They are working cooperatively to inform the intelligent development of smart multi-generational neighbourhoods. For future research, we evaluate the age-friendliness of smart multi-relationship cities using further principles. The growing growth of smart-phones with GPS and online social networks provides useful citizen involvement tools in resolving urban issues. Future research may provide more effective and user-friendly tools for assessing the age-friendly friendliness of the smart city. Thus, smartphones equipped with GPS enable citizens to enter geographical data related to the city environment into the system using any network, any-where, and at any time. This marvel empowers the procedure of evaluating and monitoring the age-friendliness of a smart city.

Acknowledgement. This research work was funded by the Smart and Health Ageing through People Engaging in supporting Systems SHAPES project, which has received funding from the European Union's Horizon 2020 research and innovation programme under grant agreement No 857159. Parts of this work have been applied in order to serve as a demonstrated solution by the Interreg Program "Greece-Cyprus 2014–2020" under the 2nd call for bilateral strategic projects of the Project with Title and acronym: "Astrological observation and natural environment- An alternative product for the development and promotion of Eastern Mediterranean geoparks" (GEOSTARS).

References

1. Sloan, J.P.: Essentials of geriatrics and aging. In Protocols in Primary Care Geri-atrics, pp. 7–12. Springer, New York (1991). https://doi.org/10.1007/978-1-4684-0388-6_2
2. Sun, F.C., Stark, L., Nguyen, A., Wong, J.A.M.E.S., Lakshminarayanan, V.A.S.U.D.E.V.A.N., Mueller, E.: Changes in accommodation with age: static and dynamic. Am. J. Optom. Physiol. Opt. **65**(6), 492–498 (1988)
3. Pirkl, J.J.: Transgenerational design: prolonging the American dream. Gen. J. Am. Soc. Aging **19**(1), 32–36 (1995)
4. Vos, J.J.: Reflections on glare. Light. Res. Technol. **35**(2), 163–175 (2003)
5. Elliott, D.B., Whitaker, D.: Changes in macular function throughout adulthood. Doc. Ophthalmol. **76**(3), 251–259 (1990)
6. Elliott, D., Whitaker, D., MacVeigh, D.: Neural contribution to spatiotemporal contrast sensitivity decline in healthy ageing eyes. Vision. Res. **30**(4), 541–547 (1990)
7. Scialfa, C.T., Adams, E.M., Giovanetto, M.A.R.K.: Reliability of the Vistech Con-trast Test System in a life-span adult sample. Opt. Vision Sci.: official publication of the American Academy of Optometry **68**(4), 270–274 (1991)
8. Scialfa, C.T., Garvey, P.M., Tyrrell, R.A., Leibowitz, H.W.: Age differences in dynamic contrast thresholds. J. Gerontol. **47**(3), P172–P175 (1992)
9. Johnson, C.A., Adams, A.J., Twelker, J.D., Quigg, J.M.: Age-related changes in the central visual field for short-wavelength-sensitive pathways. JOSA A **5**(12), 2131–2139 (1988)

10. Wijk, H., Berg, S., Sivik, L., Steen, B.: Color discrimination, color naming and color preferences in 80-year olds. Aging Clin. Exp. Res. **11**(3), 176–185 (1999). https://doi.org/10.1007/BF03399660
11. Ball, K.K., Beard, B.L., Roenker, D.L., Miller, R.L., Griggs, D.S.: Age and visual search: Expanding the useful field of view. JOSA A **5**(12), 2210–2219 (1988)
12. Edwards, J.D., et al.: The useful field of view test: normative data for older adults. Arch. Clin. Neuropsychol. **21**(4), 275–286 (2006)
13. Al-Shayea, T.K., Mavromoustakis, C.X., Batalla, J.M., Mastorakis, G.: A hybridized methodology of different wavelet transformations targeting medical images in IoT infrastructure. Measurement **148**, 106813 (2019)
14. Davis, A.C., Ostri, B., Parving, A.: Longitudinal study of hearing. Acta Otolaryngol. **111**(sup476), 12–22 (1991)
15. Pedersen, K.E., Rosenhall, U., Metier, M.B.: Changes in pure-tone thresholds in individuals aged 70–81: results from a longitudinal study. Audiology **28**(4), 194–204 (1989)
16. Fitzgibbons, P.J., Gordon-Salant, S., Barrett, J.: Age-related differences in discrimination of an interval separating onsets of successive tone bursts as a function of interval duration. J. Acoust. Soc. Am. **122**(1), 458–466 (2007)
17. Li, J.Q., et al.: Design of a continuous blood pressure measurement system based on pulse wave and ECG signals. IEEE J. Transl. Eng. Health Med. **6**, 1–14 (2018)
18. Kline, D.W., Scialfa, C.T.: Sensory and perceptual functioning: basic research and human factors implications (1997)
19. Lin, Y.H., Hsieh, S.C., Chao, C.C., Chang, Y.C., Hsieh, S.T.: Influence of aging on thermal and vibratory thresholds of quantitative sensory testing. J. Peripher. Nerv. Syst. **10**(3), 269–281 (2005)
20. Fisk, D., Charness, N., Czaja, S.J., Rogers, W.A., Sharit, J.: Designing for Older Adults. CRC Press, Boca Raton (2004)
21. Newton, R.: Balance and falls among older people. Generations **27**(1), 27–31 (2003)
22. Tideiksaar, R.: Sensory impairment and fall risk. Gen. J. Am. Soc. Aging **26**(4), 22–27 (2002)
23. Nikoloudakis, Y., Pallis, E., Mastorakis, G., Mavromoustakis, C.X., Skianis, C., Markakis, E.K.: Vulnerability assessment as a service for fog-centric ICT ecosystems: a healthcare use case. Peer-to-Peer Networking Appl. **12**(5), 1216–1224 (2019). https://doi.org/10.1007/s12083-019-0716-y
24. Easterby, R. (ed.): Anthropometry and Biomechanics: Theory and Application, vol. 16. Springer, New York (2012)
25. Salthouse, T.A.: The aging of working memory. Neuropsychology **8**(4), 535 (1994)
26. Scullin, M.K., Bugg, J.M., McDaniel, M.A., Einstein, G.O.: Prospective memory and aging: Preserved spontaneous retrieval, but impaired deactivation, in older adults. Mem. Cognit. **39**(7), 1232–1240 (2011)
27. Spaan, P.E.: Episodic and semantic memory functioning in very old age: explanations from executive functioning and processing speed theories. Cogent Psychol. **2**(1), 1109782 (2015)
28. Sweatt, J.D. (ed.): Mechanisms of Memory. Academic Press (2009)
29. McDowd, J.M., Shaw, R.J.: Attention and aging: a functional perspective (2000)
30. Burgess, N.: Spatial cognition and the brain. Ann. N. Y. Acad. Sci. **1124**(1), 77–97 (2008)
31. Beaudet, G., et al.: Spatial memory deficit across aging: current insights of the role of 5-HT7 receptors. Front. Behav. Neurosci. **8**, 448 (2015)

32. Ganchev, I., Garcia, N.M., Dobre, C., Mavromoustakis, C.X., Goleva, R. (eds.): Enhanced Living Environments: Algorithms, Architectures, Platforms, and Systems, Vol. 11369. Springer, Cham (2019). https://doi.org/10.1007/978-3-030-10752-9

33. Andreas, A., et al.: Towards an optimized security approach to IoT devices with confidential healthcare data exchange. Multimedia Tools Appl. **80**(20), 31435–31449 (2021). https://doi.org/10.1007/s11042-021-10827-x

34. Andreas, A., Mastorakis, G., Batalla, J.M., Sahalos, J.N., Pallis, E., Markakis, E.: Robust encryption to enhance IoT confidentiality for healthcare ecosystems. In: 2021 IEEE 26th International Workshop on Computer Aided Modeling and Design of Communication Links and Networks (CAMAD), pp. 1–6. IEEE, October 2021

35. Andreas, A., Mavromoustakis, C.X., Mastorakis, G., Batalla, J.M.: Network security by merging two robust tools from the mathematical firmament. In: 2021 17th International Conference on Mobility, Sensing and Networking (MSN), pp. 616–621. IEEE, December 2021

36. Andreas, A., Mavromoustakis, C.X., Mastorakis, G., Mumtaz, S., Batalla, J.M., Pallis, E.: Modified machine learning Techique for curve fitting on regression models for COVID-19 projections. In: 2020 IEEE 25th International Workshop on Computer Aided Modeling and Design of Communication Links and Networks (CAMAD), pp. 1–6. IEEE, September 2020

Application of KNN for Fall Detection on Qualcomm SoCs

Purab Nandi[✉], Apoorva Bajaj, and K. R. Anupama

Birla Institute of Technology and Science, Pilani, K.K Birla Goa Campus, Goa 403726, India
{p20200056,f20180269,anupkr}@goa.bits-pilani.ac.in

Abstract. A fall of an elderly person often leads to serious injuries, even death. Many falls occur in the home environment, and hence, a reliable fall detection system that can raise alarms immediately is a necessity. Wrist-worn accelerometer-based fall detection systems have been developed, and there are various data sets available, but the accuracy and precision have not been standardized or compared; even where comparison does exist, it has been run on GPUs. No analysis of the workability of the models and the data sets on SoCs has been previously attempted. Though over the last few years, ML and DL algorithms have been increasingly used in fall detection, and there have also been some suggestions for the use of compressed modelling, there are no concrete statistics available to form this conclusion. In this paper, we attempt to understand why ML algorithms cannot run as-is on existing SoCs; We are using Snapdragon 410c to do our analytics as it is primarily used in Biomedical and IoT applications, has low power consumption and small form factor making it ideal for wearables. In this paper, we have used KNN to prove that ML cannot be used directly on SoCs. We are using KNN as it does not have any pre-training period, and it is a very simple algorithm that gives good accuracy. In this paper, we establish the need for model and data compression for fall detection if we must use ML or DL algorithms on SOCs. We have done this with statistical analysis across different data sets.

Keywords: SoC · Wearable · IoT · KNN

1 Introduction

Medical and healthcare advancements have increased the average human lifespan to over 80 years. Geriatric healthcare hence has become vital, and regular monitoring of parameters is required. Currently, visiting or in-house nursing staff do the monitoring of various parameters. This arrangement is expensive for a significant part of society; the past decade has witnessed substantial technological advances in IoT based wearable devices, machine and deep learning; these technologies are now increasingly used in the healthcare domain. IoT-based healthcare includes tracking patients, inventory management of drugs, collection of patient samples, authentication of the patients and staff, and automated data collection and storage. IoT in the healthcare domain enables all these applications due to the availability of various wearable and non-wearable devices. These

S. Spinsante et al. (Eds.): HealthyIoT 2022, LNICST 456, pp. 148–169, 2023.
https://doi.org/10.1007/978-3-031-28663-6_12

devices are used for remote diagnosis, prognosis, and treatment. Hence advances in IoT, embedded systems and ML are the catalysts in the development of geriatric healthcare systems. Such systems are available at a reduced cost for detecting anomalies and raising timely alerts, assistance and care when required. Such a system is essential in a country like India, with a rising population of seniors residing in isolation. Some of the common concerns of the geriatric population include falls, sleep apnea, hiatus hernia, and other respiratory disorders that do not have a surgical solution, and the primary cause is frailty. Medical literature [1] also indicates that these disorders generally compound into life-threatening disorders.

Falls - According to a WHO report, there is an exponential increase in the frequency of falls with frailty and age. The elderly population in nursing homes are more susceptible to falls than those in the community. Falls usually result in recurrent falls. WHO data validates these statistics; It indicates that 40% of the falls among the elderly are recurrent falls.

Sleep Apnea - Sleep apnea is prevalent in adults and a small percentage of juveniles. Subjects suffering from sleep apnea experience periods of shallow breathing while asleep. Periods of shallow breathing or air flow reduction are called a hypopnea. This condition ultimately leads to apnea which causes breathing to stop temporarily. Both these conditions can cause clinical co-morbidity.

Hiatal Hernia -Hiatal hernia is when the stomach bulges up into the chest via an opening in the diaphragm. The muscles that separate the diaphragm from the stomach are called the hiatus. There are mainly two types of hiatus hernia (i) sliding (ii) para-esophageal.

Most elderlies suffer from the former type of hernia, which is inoperable. Hiatus hernia causes a person to exasperate their food which causes a drop in the O_2 level; SpO_2 sensors can detect the drop in O_2 level, which prevents the need for complex and costly diagnostic processes like polysomnography.

Sensors can be used to monitor the above three health conditions, and they can relay data to a smart ML-based system that can detect and predict the condition. In this paper we concentrate on fall-detections, the causes of falls are primarily categorized into internal and external. External causes of falls are due to environmental factors like slippery surfaces. Internal causes include cramps, weakness in the muscular-skeletal structure, vision impairments, chronic disorders, etc. The duration of the fall is also important. According to [2], about 40% of the individuals who fall cannot get up on their own, and about 50% who experience a long fall are likely to die within the next few months. A long-duration fall can also result in localized muscle injury, tissue damage, nerve issues, dehydration, hypothermia, pneumonia and a fear of further falls. These conditions affect the overall health of the elderly. Although numerous studies [3] related to fall detection have been out recently, several challenges still exists. These include:

(a) The lack of a comprehensive analysis of ML techniques deployed to detect falls (b) A high number of false positives (c) The low accuracy of systems that are expected to detect and correct such false positives (d) The inability of the system to detect the duration of the fall.

With technological advances in SoCs and IoT systems, wearable devices have emerged as a leading area of research in geriatric health care; the amount of data collected at homes/hospitals for the elderly is large and complex and making accurate decisions based on multiple parameters is the primary requirement for such safety-critical systems. SoCs are resource-constrained devices, whether in terms of memory, processing power or energy constraints. Hence, they cannot implement ML algorithms or Deep Neural Networks. Hence a possible solution for this is the use of model compression. This paper picks up one of the simplest ML algorithms and runs them on varying data sets of different sizes to prove that it is impossible to run even a simple ML algorithm such as KNN when the data set size is considerable. Not only is the latency high, but as the size of the data set increases, the SoC fails, indicating the non-availability of the required resources. This paper proves that ML algorithms give inaccurate, non-reliable and high latency results when run on a raw data set. Hence this paper builds a case for using model compression algorithms while using SoCs.

The paper is organized as follows: Sect. 2 talks about various IoT architectures that can be used for fall detection, Sect. 3 gives a brief overview of ML algorithms used for fall detection, Sect. 4 provides the operational details of KNN, while Sect. 5 gives the details of the dataset used for analysis, we present our results in Sect. 6, while Sect. 7 summaries and concludes this paper.

2 Architectural Models for IoT Based Fall Detection Systems with Wearable End Devices

With the growth of SoCs and its integration into IoT systems, wearable healthcare devices are now a focused area of research. This section presents four possible IoT architectural models that can be used for health care. The models vary in terms of how the data is gathered, processed and where the conversion of data to knowledge occurs.

Model A- In this architectural model, the data is collected at regular sampling intervals from the sensors that are interfaced with the wearable devices. The wearable device then transmits the raw data to the coordinator; the co-ordinator then collects the data from multiple wearables, aggregates the data and forwards the data to the cloud. The actual analysis and processing of data take place on the cloud. The sensor fusion algorithms that require combining data from multiple sensors also run on the cloud. The essential features are then extracted from the fused data and converted to health parameters using ML or DL algorithms. In this architectural model, data storage, as well as the processing of data, is done on the cloud. The data processing may be for emergency or long-term monitoring. The end devices are minimalistic and constrained in terms of processing and memory capabilities. The coordinator only acts as an aggregator of data. The focus of this architecture is on developing networking protocols that can deliver the data to the cloud with minimum latency and control overhead.

Model B –Similar to the case of model A, the wearable end device collects the raw data and transmits it to the coordinator. The coordinator aggregates the data and performs multi-sensor fusion on the raw data. The fused data is then sent to the cloud by the coordinator, the cloud performs feature extraction and converts the data to health parameters using ML/DL algorithms. In this model, while network protocols are also important, the architecture of the coordinator also needs to be carefully considered. Since sensor fusion is performed at the coordinator, the coordinator must be a powerful

SoC. The advantage of this model would be that the amount of communication between the coordinator and the cloud is reduced. This reduces the communication bandwidth requirement, but the actual conversion of data to knowledge still happens on the cloud. Model A and B may not be suitable for emergency response due to the latencies involved in communication. If the coordinator cannot connect to the cloud, any falls detected cannot immediately trigger an alarm (Figs. 1, 2, 3 and 4).

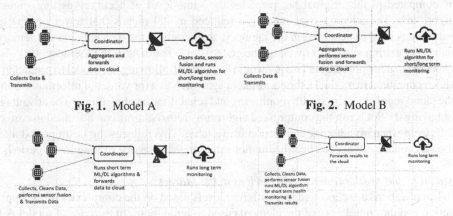

Fig. 1. Model A   **Fig. 2.** Model B

Fig. 3. Model C   **Fig. 4.** Model D

Model C- In the case of architectural model C, the wearable end device is more powerful as it not only collects data from multiple sensors but also runs sensor fusion algorithms. The wearable device then transmits these fused data to the coordinator. In many cases, the sensor fusion algorithm that runs on the wearable device is more statistical in nature. The end device in model C must be a powerful microcontroller that can run complex mathematical and thresholding algorithms. Using ML algorithms, the coordinator then converts the fused data to short-term health parameters. In case of any falls or lie-ins detected, the coordinator raises the alarm. The cloud then runs only the ML and DL algorithms that are required for long-term health monitoring and rehabilitation. In the case of model C, the end device needs to have more processing power and at the same time also be able to handle complex network algorithms to transmit the fused data to the coordinator. The latencies in communication between the end device and the coordinator still exist even though the latency in raising the alarm is considerably reduced. Here data processing is done by all elements of the IoT model. While the end device performs sensor fusion, ML/DL algorithms to extract information from the fused data is run at the coordinator while the cloud converts data into long-term health parameters.

Model D – In the case of architectural model D, the wearable device is built using a powerful SoC as it is responsible for collecting data from multiple sensors, fusing it, and running ML and DL algorithms to detect/predict falls. This requires considerable processing power; The wearable device is required to collect and clean the data, perform sensor fusion, extract the required features and then convert the data into information using a complex ML/DL algorithm. Though SoCs have considerably advanced to handle complex biomedical applications, they are still constrained in terms of the amount of memory available, energy consumed and form factor. As the device is wearable, the form factor must be very less. At the same time, power consumption must also be limited. Heat dissipation is another issue that is common in wearable devices. Running complex processing algorithms will cause the processor to expend more heat. Hence, running ML, DL, or deep neural networks widely used in IoT-based health services is very difficult. Over the last couple of years, research in model compression of ML and DL algorithms has gained traction. The goal of model compression is to achieve a model that is simplified as compared to the original but provides the same level of accuracy as the original algorithms. The advantage of running a reduced model means that fewer or smaller parameters need to be stored in the memory, as not only is the data resident in memory, but the operating system, as well as the code, is also resident in the memory. It is also expected that the processing latency would be reduced, allowing the model to predict in a shorter duration. In model D, the coordinator again acts as a forwarder of information, and the cloud runs long-term health monitoring and rehabilitation algorithms. The advantage of having the SoCs run the compressed algorithms is that alarms can be raised in case of falls even when no network connection is available. This reduces the lie-in period after the fall, reducing complex health situations that might arise due to long lie-in periods.

Model D and Available Wearable Devices in the Market

IoT applications are classified into different levels based on the complexity of the application and the complexity of the elements used to build them. In the case of model A,B and C described in this section, data storage and analytics is not done on the wearable device. Health monitoring systems usually collect a large amount of data from multiple sensors. The size of the data is large and also requires complex data analytics. Hence using the usual classification of IoT systems, the data storage and analytics must be primarily performed on the cloud. While this model works well for long-term health monitoring and rehabilitation, it will not be suitable for emergency services. In our suggested model D, we store some of the data and run the complex data analytics on them to handle an emergency such as falls; hence each end device has a very powerful SoC at its core. We plan to use SoCs such as Qualcomm Snapdragon 410c/820c/wear 4100 series that are built explicitly for biomedical applications. Running ML/DL applications especially requires high processing power. Hence if the analytics for emergency care must be performed on wearable devices, we need to use compressed ML algorithms.

We have reviewed multiple fall detection-based systems [4] available commercially and under theoretical research. In the following subsection, we give a brief overview of such fall detection systems.

Commercially Available Systems and Their Applications

Apple watch SE or series 4 [5] and above can detect hard falls. These services are enabled by default if you are above 55 years of age and are available as an optional application for those between 18 to 55. The "apple watch fall detection app" can help connect users to emergency services while sending messages to their emergency contacts. Apple Watch can detect only hard falls. It uses accelerometer and gyroscope data to detect a fall. It uses the impact acceleration and the resultant wrist trajectory for fall detection. In order to detect falls, it uses thresholding technology on the data, and no ML/DL algorithms are run on the wearable system. Apple Watch also detects if a person is immobile for 60 s, it then begins a 30 s counter that starts an audio alert. The audio alert keeps getting louder until emergency services press "cancel". Despite the availability of such features, experimental data show the accuracy is only 4.7%, it has a false-negative rate of 95.3% and an interesting point is also that Apple watches are better at detecting forward falls than sideways falls because the wrist movement in sideways fall is equivalent to lying down in bed.

Another smart wearable device available is the "Unali Kanega" watch [6], another wrist-based device available for fall detection. It also makes use of accelerometer data to detect falls. The Unali watch is unique because the user can change the battery while still wearing the watch. This is a useful feature since falls may occur when the user removes his watch to charging.

There is also the Phoenix watch available which has an app called WellB Medical Alert plus that sends out the GPS location of the fallen person as long as he presses the button.

Other than the wearable systems available commercially, there are also applications which can run on the mobile. The summary of the applications and their capability is listed in the table given below. All the applications require that a user either presses a button or uses some form of an audio alert. The application will only provide the GPS location of the person. (Wherever GPS+ is mentioned in the table, it also uses Wi-Fi information to detect the person's position).

Other than these, there are also the popular "fall call lite application" [7] which usually runs on the Watch Operating Systems. Here the user must press a button and call for help when he falls. These applications are not very popular as they require that the person is still conscious and able to raise an alert.

The Wearable Devices Under Research
[8] talks about a smart vest that can monitor respiratory and physical activities. The M-health platform [9] described as part of the "Frail" project has a smart vest, fall sensors, and a smartwatch. The sensing platform aims to address the continuous monitoring of vital signs relevant to frail users and detecting and alerting falls. The smart watch worn by the user acts as the gateway to the platform, gathering data from sensors and receiving events and remainders introduced by caregivers.

Since the smartwatch is responsible for communication with the frail servers, the end devices, the sensing platforms, need only to send the sensor data. Hence this falls under model C of the IoT architecture described in Sect. 2. For fall detection, mainly accelerometer-based devices are used. Also, after the accelerometer detects the fall, the smartwatch expects the wearer to confirm he/she has fallen. If the user confirms the fall, the smartwatch sends the event to the frail servers back and then triggers a preconfigured procedure. The sensor module used is a tri-axial accelerometer, and the processing module is a PIC18 F2431 Microcontroller which uses a thresholding method to detect falls. The sensors are placed as an adhesive patch on the skin of the lower back. Again, this system does not use multiple sensor data or any machine learning algorithm to detect falls.

Table 1. The summary of commercially available wearables

Product	Automaticfall detection	Location capability	Battery life
GreatCall *Lively Mobile Plus*	Yes	GPS	1–3 days
Philips Lifeline *GoSafe 2*	Yes	GPS+	2–3 days
Medical Guardian *Active Guardian* (rebranded version of the Freeus *Belle+*)	Yes	GPS+	up to 5 days
LifeFone *At home, On-the-Go GPS, Voice in Pendant* (rebranded version of the Freeus *Belle+*)	Yes	GPS+	up to 5 days (30 days if no fall detection capability)
LifeFone *At home, On-the-Go GPS* (rebranded version of the MobileHelp *Duo*)	Yes	GPS	1 day (mobile base station) pendant: long
MobileHelp *Duo*	Yes	GPS	1 day (mobile base station) pendant: 18 months
Medical Guardian *Mini Guardian*	Yes	GPS+	up to 5 days

Further research analysis shows that most fall detection systems use Model A, while the rest may use Model B, where sensor fusion is done on the coordinating device. This will be the first attempt to build a wearable SoC device that runs compressed ML\DL algorithms that provide auto alerts for emergency help.

3 Machine Learning

ML [10] is a technique that applies mathematical models to data sets to analyze, classify and convert data into knowledge. There are three types of ML algorithms.

1. Supervised – In supervised learning, the input data is classified apriori using a training data set; any new data is automatically classified into one of the input types, some of the algorithms include KNN [11], Naïve Bayes [12], Decision trees [13], Linear Regression [14], SVM [15].
2. Unsupervised – In unsupervised learning, the ML algorithm recognizes a pattern on its own from a given data set, some of the common algorithms include K-Means clustering [16], Classification rules [17], Hidden Markov model [18], Neural Networks [19].

3. Reinforced -This algorithm allows the system to adapt its behavior based on feedback from the environment.

In the case of fall detection, binary classification is used to convert an activity into a fall or ADL. The diagram given below shows how the ML model is built.
In each category of ML, there are several algorithms, as shown in Fig. 5.

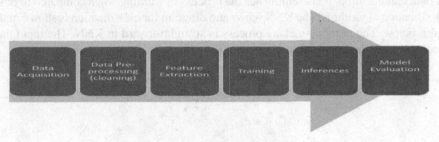

Fig. 5. Schematic of ML Model

For fall detection, several ML algorithms are currently being used. Commonly used algorithms are Logical Regression, Naïve Bayes, SVM, K Nearest Neighbor and Random Forest. Among these algorithms, this paper concentrates on the KNN algorithm. We had earlier run multiple ML algorithms for fall detection. The AUC/ROC curve for them is shown in the figure below.

The algorithms were run on the data set that we had collected. The dataset had over 70k points, of which 70% was used for training; and 30% was used as test data. KNN has a good AUC score of 0.971, performing as well as SVM. We have used KNN to analyze the latencies involved in the ML algorithm as the accuracies of KNN are good, and KNN does not require any pre-training until a query is raised. Hence KNN is the best model to understand the effect of implementing ML on SoCs as there will be no heavy pre-training required, unlike the other algorithms. Though Naïve-Bayes is easier to implement. Its AUC score is only 0.825, which is very low when compared to KNN (Fig. 6).

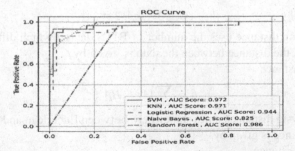

Fig. 6. AUC/ROC curve of ML algorithms for fall detection

4   K Nearest Neighbor Classification Algorithm (KNN)

The KNN algorithm [20] is a general classification algorithm that uses Nearest Neighbor rules to classify data. It compares the input data with K samples with the same class label, finds the nearest one, and classifies the input data accordingly. It differs from the Nearest Neighbor algorithm in that, instead of a single neighbor, it takes K nearest neighbor in the decision-making process. This allows the KNN algorithm to utilize more information for data classification. It also eliminates the process of learning when compared to other classification algorithms. The KNN schematic diagram for classification is shown in the figure below. The decision-making process is straightforward in KNN. The input data is compared to the sample class close to it (Fig. 7).

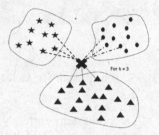

Fig. 7. Classification Schematic for k = 3

The classification is done based on the distance metric, as shown in the figure above. There are multiple methods available to calculate the distance in KNN. The most commonly used methods are (a) Euclidean, (b) Manhattan, (c) Hamming (d) Minkowski [21].

The Euclidean distance is calculated using the formula given below.
Euclidian distance

$$d = \sqrt{(x_2 - x_1)^2 - (y_2 - y_1)^2} \tag{1}$$

The Manhattan distance is the distance between two points measured along the axis at right angles and uses the following formulae for calculating the distance.
Manhattan distance

$$d = |x_2 - x_1| + |y_2 - y_1| \tag{2}$$

The Hamming distance uses the number of BITS dataset which differ between the two-binary data, the distance between the data is given by
Hamming distance

$$d = \sum |A_i - B_i| \tag{3}$$

The Minkowski distance comes somewhere between Euclidean and Hamming. The Minkowski distance is given by
Minkowski distance

$$d = \sum_{i=1}^{n} (x_i - y_i)^{\frac{1}{p}} \tag{4}$$

5   Dataset and Data Preparation

The size of the data set, the data collection methodology used, the nature of the sensors, and the sampling rate affect the model's output. Research in fall detection has advanced over the last few years due to the increase in the elderly population who live alone. Multiple fall data sets are available, and various data sets [22] have been analyzed in detail. When coming to falls, the sensors used for fall detection can be (a) Biological, (b) IMU, (c) Image (d) Ambient sensors. While the first two fall under the wearable sensor category, the latter are non-wearable. Biological sensors might be heartrate sensors, GSR sensors, SpO_2 sensors or sensors based on the previous health history of the person. IMU sensors include a 3D accelerometer and gyroscope. Image sensors are monochrome/RGB/Thermal cameras/IR cameras, which detect falls. Ambient sensors are usually placed around the entire room occupied by the elderly. This includes radar and acoustic sensors, which are used for detecting falls.

Wearable sensors are preferred because they can follow the elderly through their entire daily routine. Multiple wearable sensors are available, primarily IMU-based sensors, most of which use 3D accelerometers. 80% of the data set available currently have waist-worn accelerometer sensors. Some supplement the waist-worn sensors by placing the sensors on the thigh or leg of the sensor. Few data sets place sensors all over the torso. Wearing sensors on the waist and the torso can be highly uncomfortable for the elderly as these sensors have to be worn for the entire day. In this paper, we focus on wrist-worn sensors as we strongly believe a wrist sensor is more convenient for an elderly user, and the sensor data can constantly be augmented appropriately using mathematical models.

Furthermore, there are multiple fitness bands available in the market that provide IMU and heart rate, blood pressure, and oxygen levels, and these devices can very quickly be adapted for fall detection. Fitness bands come with their own SoCs, so we believe we can adapt ML algorithms to be run locally on the device and the data to be stored locally for short-term health emergencies such as falls. We examined multiple datasets which used 3D accelerometers and looked mainly at data sets where the sensors were worn on the wrist. Among these, Smartwatch, SmartFall and Notch datasets are available publicly, so we used them. We also collected data using ten volunteers wearing a TIC watch (BITS dataset).

Data Collection Methodology for BITS Dataset
We gathered our data using ten volunteers wearing a TIC watch which included a 3-axis accelerometer, 3-axis magnetometer, 3-axis gyroscope and optical heart rate sensor.

Experiments were performed in a controlled environment in 20 different ADL/fall activity simulations, such as walking, running, climbing stairs, abrupt movements, and various types of falls. Using a TIC Watch, data were collected at four samples/second, the maximum possible frequency.

The volunteers were aged between the ages of 20–22 years. Their height ranged from 5'1" to 5'8", and weight from 40 kg to 75 kg.

Experiments were performed across 20 different ADL/fall activity simulations, such as walking, running, climbing stairs, and abrupt movements. The volunteers simulated the following activities: (a) Walking slowly (b) Walking quickly (c) Jogging (d) Climbing up and down a flight of stairs (e) Slowly sitting on a chair, waiting a moment, and standing up slowly (f) Quickly sitting on a chair, waiting a moment, and standing up quickly (g) Trying to transition from sitting to standing position but collapsing midway (h)Transitioning from sitting to lying and back, slowly (i) Transitioning from sitting to lying and back, quickly (j) Transitioning from sideways position to one's back while lying down (k) Standing, about to sit down, and getting up (l) Stumbling while walking (m) Slowly jumping without falling (n) Swinging hand (o) Falls – forward, backward, left lateral, right lateral (p) Grabbing while falling (q) Spinning fall.

To collect the data, the TIC watch was programmed to collect the data and send it via the user interface to the system. The data was automatically moved into a.csv file. The user interface of the software had buttons for every type of activity that was performed, so the corresponding button was selected before performing a particular activity. This enabled automatic labelling of the dataset as it got stored.

Samples on IMU and heart rate were collected during 14 ADLs and 6 falls, with each activity/fall, repeated twice. All activities were conducted at the BITS Pilani, K K Birla Goa campus. The falls were simulated in a controlled environment. The anechoic chamber at BITS Pilani, K K Birla Goa campus was used for this purpose. The chamber, 4.5 m × 2.2 m × 2.5 m, is padded with NRL USA standard 8093 complying material on all four walls, the floor, and the ceiling. This padding provided the necessary shock absorption capabilities to protect volunteers from harm during the experimentation.

The volunteer's rebound and residual movements after a fall activity were also considered to ensure that the data set also contains post-fall values of the IMU and heart rate parameters. Hence for falls, the data collection was stopped not immediately but a few seconds after the actual event occurred, during which time the volunteers performed post-fall movements such as rolling over and attempting to get up. The data set generated had, in total, over 110,000 lines about the ADLs as mentioned above and falls.

In case of the BITS data set though we collected data using a 3 axes accelerometer, magnetometer and gyroscope as well as an optical heart rate sensor, we used only the data from 3 axes accelerometer to study the accuracies over the other data sets. This changed the number of data points from 110,000 to 47,656.

Data preparation for SmartFall, Smartwatch and Notch

Smartwatch Dataset [23]- Smartwatch had 7 subjects with the age range of 21 to 55 who perform 971 different activities. Each data was collected at a sample rate of 31 Hz. In order to match it with our data set we downscale it to 20 kHz using the python scipy 1.2.3 package overall there were 34,019 data points.

Notch Dataset [24]- Notch data set have only 7 subjects in the ages ranging from 20–35. Overall notch had 10,645 data points; the data set was also collected at 31 Hz which was eventually downscaled to 20 Hz to match our data set.

SmartFall Dataset [25] - Smartfall had more subjects (14) covering a wider age range of 21 to 60, covering 1027 activities and 92,780 data points. Again, as in case of Smartwatch and Notch, we down sample the smartwatch data to 20 Hz.

Fused Dataset - We also fused the data set of SmartFall, Smartwatch and Notch as all 3 of them use the same accelerometer and a sampling rate of 31.25 Hz. This gave us overall 2496 activities extended over 28 subjects in the age range of 20–60. We combined the data set as we wanted to understand the effect of the size of the data set on the performance of the ML algorithm, especially in terms of latency, as we implemented it on the Qualcomm Snapdragon 410c SoC.

A summary of all data sets is shown in the Table 2.

We did not combine the BITS data set in the fused data set as a completely different accelerometer was used to collect data. The data ranges were completely different, and the ML algorithms would have given entirely incorrect results. We did not upscale or downscale the data because no mathematical relationship could be derived from the data sets due to the use of entirely different sensors. Any min-max scale or thresholding would have required that we examine over 100,000 data points to look for similarities between various falls and non-falls events. This would have required a considerable performance and computational complexity tradeoff (Table 1).

Table 2. Summary of datasets used in this paper

Dataset	Activities	Data points	Test subjects	Age
BITS	3000	47,656	10	20–22
Notch	698	10,645	7	20–35
SmartWatch	771	34,019	7	21–55
SmartFall	1027	92,780	14	21–60
Fused	2496	137,444	28	20–60

6   Results and Discussions

To understand the working of ML on an SoC, we choose to experiment with KNN as the ML model. As mentioned in Sect. 4, the primary advantage of KNN is that no pre-training is required until a query is raised. As described in Sect. 5, we worked with multiple data sets such as a Smartwatch, Smartfall and Notch. This was to understand the effect of data collection and results of the data set on the accuracy of the ML model. Furthermore, to understand the limitations of the data set size, that the SoC could work while we used the clean data set from the Smartwatch and Smartfall and Notch all of them down sample to 20 Hz; we also used the data collected by us in both the raw and clean format. Data cleaning or statistical analysis of data is generally performed on the cloud. If we collect data and send it to the cloud for cleaning, the network latency remains; hence, running the ML algorithms on the SoC has no benefit. Hence the cleaning of the data should also happen on the SoC itself. When we use raw data, the SoC is unable to proceed further. More details are given below in this section.While analyzing the various datasets and the effect of running the algorithm on an SoC, we varied the values of k from 1-to 200. In some cases, we have looked at a narrower data window with k values varying between 17–69 because that is where the maximum variation was observed. We also ran the accuracy for three different distance equations, Euclidian, Minkowski and Manhattan. When we attempted to run the algorithm with Hamming distance, the accuracies were considerably lower. As most of our data is 64-bit floating-point format and there are minimal variations in mantissa values, Hamming does not work well with the kind of data set we are using. We also analyzed the latencies of the various datasets. We ran the algorithms for varying values of k on Apple M1 systems and Qualcomm Snapdragon 410c. We ran the algorithm on the M1 system as a single thread since the SoC also runs the algorithm as a single thread. The apple M1 pro was running at 3.22 Ghz, and the 410C SoC was running at 2.40 GHz.

The plots of our various results are given below:

Figures 8 and 9 give the accuracy and latencies of Smartwatch on M1 pro.

Figures 10 and 11 give the accuracy and latency of Smartwatch on Qualcomm 410c.

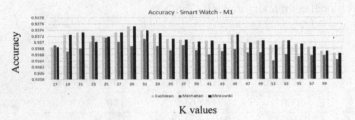

Fig. 8. Accuracy of Smartwatch dataset on Apple M1 pro

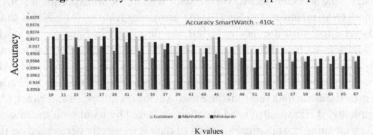

Fig. 9. Latency on Smartwatch dataset on Apple M1 pro

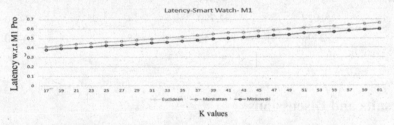

Fig. 10. Accuracy of Smartwatch dataset on Qualcomm 410c

Analysis of Smartwatch Dataset Results

In the case of Smartwatch, there are 771 data taken from 7 subjects over ages 21 to 55. The details are given in Sect. 6. The best results were obtained at a k value of 29 for

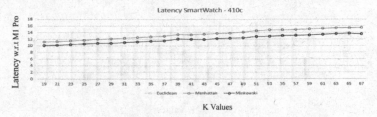

Fig. 11. Latency on Smartwatch dataset on Qualcomm 410c

both Euclidean and Minkowski, while Manhattan gave its best result at a slightly lower value of k = 23. This is a trend that can be observed over various datasets that Manhattan gives higher accuracies at a lower value of k; this is because of the way the distance is calculated in the case of Manhattan, which is the sum of the absolute difference of the cartesian co-ordinates of the data. It can be seen from the latency plots that the SoCs take about 10.5 s in case of the highest accuracy for both Euclidean and Minkowski are about 11.75 s for Manhattan.

The accuracy of Minkowski (93.7519%) and Euclidian (93.7519%) is slightly higher than that of Manhattan (93.7213%). Where as in the case of M1 Pro, the time taken is 0.45 s for all the algorithms. The data sampling rate in case of all our data is 20 Hz, meaning we collect a sample every 0.25 s and if the time taken to run the algorithm is between 10 to 12 s, even at a frequency of 2.4 GHz, and with a simplistic ML algorithm such as KNN, it is not possible to run an ML algorithm realtime on the SoC. The number of data points on Smartwatch is 34,019. Though it covers only 771 activities. The latencies required on the SoC are extremely high.

Analysis of Smartfall Dataset Results
In the case of Smartfall size of the data set is 92,780 data points covering 1027 activities. The best performance for Euclidian and Minkowski is obtained at a k value of 25 and in the case of Manhattan at a k value of 21. As in the previous 2 cases, the best performance of Manhattan (93.5186%) is slightly lower than that of Euclidian (93.5312%) and Minkowski (93.5312%). The latencies, as expected, are higher as the data set size is more extensive. Euclidian and Minkowski's peak performance, the latency incurred by M1 pro is 0.65, and in the case of Manhattan, it is 0.7. The latencies in the case of 410c for Euclidean and Minkowski is 21 s and 23 s for Manhattan.

Figures 12 and 13 give the accuracy and latency of Smartfall on M1 pro.

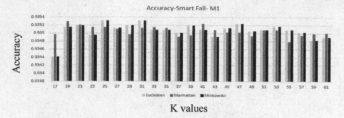

Fig. 12. Accuracy of Smartfall dataset on Apple M1 pro

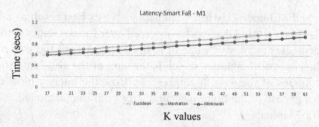

Fig. 13. Latency on Smartfall dataset on Apple M1 pro

Figures 14 and 15 give the accuracy and latency of Smartfall on Qualcomm 410c.

Analysis of Notch Dataset Results
The Notch data set has 10,645 data points covering overall 698 activities. This is by far the smallest data set that we have used. The accuracy of the Notch data set is at k = 35 for both Euclidean and Minkowski; in the case of Manhattan, the maximum accuracy is observed at k = 31. The latencies of the Notch dataset, in the case of both Apple M1 processor and 410c, are slightly lesser as the dataset size is also lesser. In the case of Euclidean and Minkowski at the peak performance, the latency on the M1 processor for the Notch data set is at 0.4 s, and for Manhattan, it is at 0.45 s.

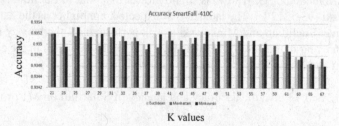

Fig. 14. Accuracy of Smartfall dataset on Qualcomm 410c

While in the case of 410c at the peak performance, the latencies are 10 s for Minkowski and Euclidian and 12 s for Manhattan. In the case of the Notch data set as well, the accuracy of Manhattan (91.8365%) is slightly lesser than that of Euclidean (91.8485%) and Minkowski (91.8485%).

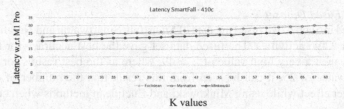

Fig. 15. Latency on Smartfall dataset on Qualcomm 410c

Figures 16 and 17 give the accuracy and latency of Notch on Apple M1 pro.

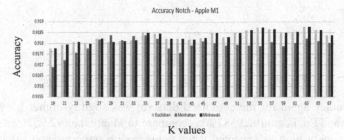

Fig. 16. Accuracy of Notch dataset on Apple M1 pro

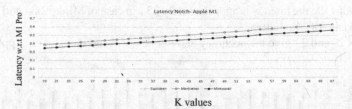

Fig. 17. Latency on Notch dataset on Apple M1 pro

Figures 18 and 19 give the accuracy and latency of Notch on Qualcomm 410c.

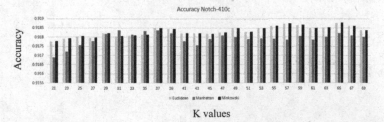

Fig. 18. Accuracy of Notch dataset on Qualcomm 410c

Analysis of Fused Dataset

As described in Sect. 5, we fused the data of Smartfall, Smartwatch and Notch generating 137,444 for 2,496 activities. The fused data set gave the best accuracy for Minkowski and Euclidean at a very high value of k = 49, where as the best results for Manhattan was at a k value of 25, it can be seen from this result that the number of data points have a bigger effect while using Minkowski and Euclidean methods when compared to Manhattan.

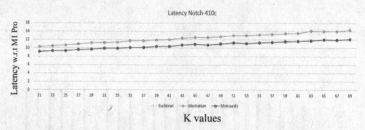

Fig. 19. Latency on Notch dataset on Qualcomm 410c

The accuracy again for the combined data set was slightly higher for Minkowski (92.9587%) and Euclidean(92.9587%)as compare to Manhattan(92.9526%). The latencies are extremely high as expected when compared to previous non fused data sets. For M1 pro, for the peak value of accuracy is at 0.75s and in case of Minkowski and Euclidean and for Manhattan the peak accuracy is observed at 0.8 s.

In case of 410c the latency is approximately 23 s in case of Minkowski and Euclidean and 24 s in case of Manhattan.

Figures 20 and 21 give the accuracy and latency of fused data-set on Apple M1 pro.

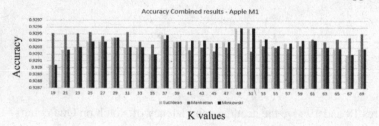

Fig. 20. Accuracy of combined dataset on Apple M1 Pro

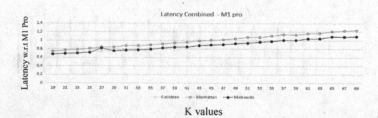

Fig. 21. Latency on combined dataset on Apple M1 Pro

Figures 22 and 23 give the accuracy and latency of combined dataset on Qualcomm 410c.

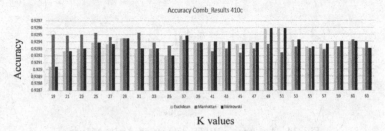

Fig. 22. Accuracy of combined dataset on Qualcomm 410c

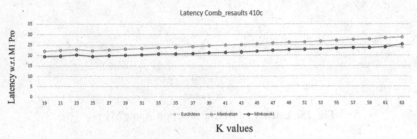

Fig. 23. Latency of combined dataset on Qualcomm 410c

BITS Data Set

In the BITS data set, we have 47,656 data points covering 20 activities. The peak accuracy of the BITS data set is obtained at 27 for all 3. The difference here is in the case of Manhattan, we get a better performance of 85.4701% compared to Minkowski (82.906%) and Euclidian (82.906%). The latencies obtained in the case of the BITS data set are slightly lesser, with the latency being 0.002 s at k = 27 for Manhattan and Minkowski, whereas it is at 0.003s for Euclidean. On Apple M1 processor. In the case of Euclidian and Minkowski, the peak latency is 0.044 s at peak performance for Euclidian and Minkowski and 0.048 for Manhattan. It can also be seen that the latency values do not increase with an increase in k. One of the reasons we could get from the data set was that the age of the subjects was almost the same, varying between 20–22 years, with none having any history of illness or falls. Hence the accuracies are lower, and latencies are lesser. As described in Sect. 5, the BITS data set, other than the accelerometer data, also has gyroscope data, heart rate, and a few other parameters. When KNN was used with all these sensors, we obtained a peak accuracy of approx. 91%, which is comparable with other data sets. The accuracy of results also depends upon the accuracy of the accelerometer used, details of which are provided in Sect. 5. Also, as all the subjects were in the same age range, therefore there is very little difference in acceleration values in terms of fall and non-fall values.

Figure 24 and 25 give the accuracy and latency of BITS dataset on Apple M1 pro Figures 26 and 27 give the accuracy and latency of BITS dataset on Qualcomm 410c.

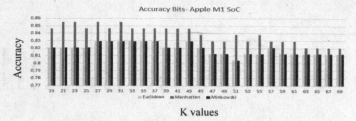

Fig. 24. Accuracy of BITS dataset on Apple M1pro

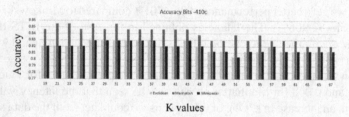

Fig. 25. Latency on BITS dataset on Apple M1 pro

Looking at the varying data sets, we can draw the following conclusions: (i) The accuracy increases with the size of training data (ii) The latencies are very high as the amount of data collected is more (iii) Statistical analysis must be performed before running the ML algorithm on the dataset. (iv) It is impossible to run ML algorithms on the SoC.

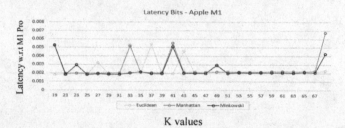

Fig. 26. Accuracy of BITS dataset on Qualcomm 410c

KNN, also considered an algorithm that does not require much pre-training, is one of the simplest algorithms to give accuracies above 90%, even with 10,000 data points requiring latencies more significant than 8 s. Hence there is a need to run compressed ML algorithms on a compressed data set. (v) When we try running the algorithm on raw data set without statistical analysis, 410c repeatedly kills the process as it cannot handle large data.

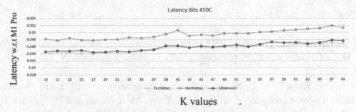

Fig. 27. Latency on BITS dataset on Qualcomm 410c

7 Summary and Conclusions

Deep learning is currently being used for fall detection. DL techniques applied on the Smartwatch, Smartfall and Notch data set gave accuracies in the range of 98.2%, 99.6% and 99%, respectively, while using CNN [26]. Some papers [27] claim RNN can be implemented on STM 32, which is built using ARM cortex M4 and the deep learning algorithms take approximately 1 s for execution. However, the pre-trained and the data set size used was only 22,321 data points. Some data were alert or pre-fall data, and the rest were fall data. The model was pre-trained to detect between pre-falls and falls, giving an accuracy of about 75%. The paper concentrates on reducing energy and power consumption rather than improving accuracy. When we ran the ML algorithm on STM 32 with the BITS data set, which has around 3000 activities and 47,656 data points, we got an accuracy of 77%. This shows that ML or DL algorithms do not converge well on microcontrollers. That is why we have moved on to SoCs.

Even in the case of SoCs though the accuracy is better, it is not possible to run uncleaned test data on the model, as we had seen with our raw test data, where the process was repeatedly killed before we applied statistical methods to derive the mean, median, max and min values after which the IMU data gave us an accuracy of around 85% while using KNN. When heart rate and gyroscope data were added to the dataset, KNN gave us an approximate accuracy of 91%. This was all achieved using Python Scikit tools. Our results show that the accuracy increases as the size of the data set increases, even with an algorithm such as KNN. If we use Model D as suggested in Sect. 2, where the ML algorithms for Fall detection are going to run on the SoC itself, it also becomes necessary to clean data, and perform sensor fusion on the SoC itself. This will take high latency on the SoC and also consume an equal amount of power. Hence, data and model compression techniques are needed if we use an extensive data set while using ensemble ML or RNN techniques. We prefer RNN as a DL technique because RNN works well with time-series data. In this paper, we have demonstrated that using SoCs to run ML algorithms is not possible. Even when running KNN, we had observed latencies in terms of seconds; hence, we need to use compressed models, and hence we have firmly established in this paper, that there is a need to use compressed models for wrist-based model D smart bands/watches. In this paper, we chose to use accelerometer data as most of the available smartwatches and smartphones are already equipped with 3-axes accelerometers. In our future work, we propose to augment this data set with biological parameters such as heart rate, SpO_2 and Galvanic skin response sensors employing RNN-based model compression algorithms.

References

1. World Population Ageing: 1950–2050. https://www.agc.org/ruralaging/world/ageingo.html
2. Tinetti, M.E.: Clinical practice: preventing falls in elderly persons. N. Engl. J. Med. **348**(1), 42–49 (2003)
3. Hausdorff, J.M., Rios, D.A., Edelberg, H.K.: Gait variability and fall risk in community-living older adults: a 1-year prospective study. Arch. Phys. Med. Rehabil. **82**(8), 1050–1056 (2001)
4. Thakur, N., Han, C.Y.: A study of fall detection in assisted living: identifying and improving the optimal machine learning method. J. Sens. Actuator Netw. **10**, 39 (2021). https://doi.org/10.3390/jsan10030039
5. Apple watch user guide. https://documents.4rgos.it
6. Kanega, U.: watch user guide. https://unaliwear.com
7. Fall call lite application documentation. https://www.fallcall.com/apps/FallCall-Lite
8. Naranjo-Hernández, D., Talaminos-Barroso, A., Reina-Tosina, J., et al.: Smart vest for respiratory rate monitoring of COPD patients based on non-contact capacitive sensing. Sens. (Basel). **18**(7), 2144 (2018). Published 3 Jul 2018. https://doi.org/10.3390/s18072144
9. Calvillo-Arbizu, J., Naranjo-Hernández, D., Barbarov-Rostán, G., Talaminos-Barroso, A., Roa-Romero, L.M., Reina-Tosina, J.: A sensor-based mhealth platform for remote monitoring and intervention of frailty patients at home. Int. J. Environ. Res. Public Health. **18**(21), 11730 (2021). Published 8 Nov 2021. https://doi.org/10.3390/ijerph182111730
10. Ramachandran, A., Karuppiah, A.: A survey on recent advances in wearable fall detection systems. BioMed. Res. Int. 2167160, 17 (2020). https://doi.org/10.1155/2020/2167160
11. Alpaydin, E.: Voting over multiple condensed nearest neighbors. Artif. Intell. Rev. 115–132 (1997)
12. Vembandasamy, K., Sasipriya, R., Deepa, E.: Heart diseases detection using Naive Bayes algorithm. IJISET – Int. J. Innov. Sci. Eng. Tech. **2**(9) (2015). ISSN 2348 – 7968
13. Hosmer, D.W., Lemeshow, S.L.: Applied Logistic Regression, 2nd edn. Wiley-Interscience, Hoboken, NJ (2000)
14. Breiman, L., Friedman, J.H., Olshen, R.A., Stone, C.J.: Classification and Regression Trees (1st ed.). Routledge (1984). https://doi.org/10.1201/9781315139470
15. Liu, S.H., Cheng, W.C.: Fall detection with the support vector machine during scripted and continuous unscripted activities. Sens. (Basel) **12**(9), 12301–12316 (2012). https://doi.org/10.3390/s120912301. Epub 2012 Sep 7. PMID: 23112713; PMCID: PMC3478840
16. Nho, Y.H., Lim, J.G., Kwon, D.S.: Cluster-analysis-based user-adaptive fall detection using fusion of heart rate sensor and accelerometer in a wearable device. IEEE Access, 1 (2020). https://doi.org/10.1109/ACCESS.2020.2969453
17. Gøeg, K.R., Cornet, R., Andersen, S.K.: Clustering clinical models from local electronic health records based on semantic similarity. J. Biomed. Inform. **54**, 294–304 (2015). https://doi.org/10.1016/j.jbi.2014.12.015ISSN 1532–0464
18. Yoon, B.J.: Hidden Markov models and their applications in biological sequence analysis. Curr. Genomics **10**(6), 402–415 (2009). https://doi.org/10.2174/138920209789177575. PMID:20190955;PMCID:PMC2766791
19. Wang, G., Liu, Z., Li, Q.: Fall detection with neural networks. In: 2019 IEEE International Flexible Electronics Technology Conference (IFETC), pp. 1–7 (2019). https://doi.org/10.1109/IFETC46817.2019.9073718
20. Xing, W., Bei, Y.: Medical health big data classification based on KNN classification algorithm. IEEE Access **8**, 28808–28819 (2020). https://doi.org/10.1109/ACCESS.2019.2955754
21. Chomboon, K., Chujai, P., Teerarassammee, P., Kerdprasop, K., Kerdprasop, N.: An Empirical Study of Distance Metrics for k-Nearest Neighbor Algorithm, pp. 280–285 (2015). https://doi.org/10.12792/iciae2015.051

22. Kraft, D., Srinivasan, K., Bieber, G.: Deep learning based fall detection algorithms for embedded systems, smartwatches, and IoT devices using accelerometers. Technologies **8**, 72 (2020). https://doi.org/10.3390/technologies8040072

23. SmartWatch dataset. https://userweb.cs.txstate.edu/~hn12/data/SmartFallDataSet/SmartWatch/

24. Notch dataset. https://userweb.cs.txstate.edu/~hn12/data/SmartFallDataSet/notch/Notch_Dataset_Wrist/

25. SmartFall dataset. https://userweb.cs.txstate.edu/~hn12/data/SmartFallDataSet/SmartFall/

26. Santos, G.L., Endo, P.T., Monteiro, K.H.D.C., Rocha, E.D.S., Silva, I., Lynn, T.: Accelerometer-based human fall detection using convolutional neural networks. Sensors **19**, 1644 (2019). https://doi.org/10.3390/s19071644

27. Farsi, M.: Application of ensemble RNN deep neural network to the fall detection through IoT environment. Alexandria Eng. J. **60**(1), 199–211 (2021). SSN 1110–0168, https://doi.org/10.1016/j.aej.2020.06.056

Assessment of Human Activity Classification Algorithms for IoT Devices

Gianluca Ciattaglia⑩, Linda Senigagliesi⑩, and Ennio Gambi$^{(\boxtimes)}$⑩

Università Politecnica delle Marche, 60131 Ancona, Italy
{g.ciattaglia,l.senigagliesi,e.gambi}@univpm.it

Abstract. Human activity classification is assuming great relevance in many fields, including the well-being of the elderly. Many methodologies to improve the prediction of human activities, such as falls or unexpected behaviors, have been proposed over the years, exploiting different technologies, but the complexity of the algorithms requires the use of processors with high computational capabilities. In this paper different deep learning techniques are compared in order to evaluate the best compromise between recognition performance and computational effort with the aim to define a solution that can be executed by an IoT device, with a limited computational load. The comparison has been developed considering a dataset containing different types of activities related to human walking obtained from an automotive Radar. The procedure requires a pre-processing of the raw data and then the feature extraction from range-Doppler maps. To obtain reliable results different deep learning architectures and different optimizers are compared, showing that an accuracy of more than 97% is achieved with an appropriate selection of the network parameters.

Keywords: Automotive radar · Deep learning · Human activities · IoT

1 Introduction

Automatic human activity classification is an active research field with applications in various contexts, such as smart monitoring, video retrieval, ambient assisted living, surveillance, etc. Mainstream techniques rely on multiple sensors placed in different parts of the human body [23], on sensors of smartphones and wearable devices (such as wristbands and watches) [25], while contactless technologies are assuming a growing relevance, thanks to their ability to provide constant monitoring without the need of placing sensors in precise positions. Among these methodologies, Radar technology has been recently applied to identify people on the basis of their gait characteristics [16,21] and gestures recognition [15,22].

Activity classification is usually performed by applying machine learning and deep learning techniques. The rise of convolutional neural networks (CNN) has resulted in the development of categorization networks such as AlexNet [12] and VGG [18]. AlexNet that is the first DNN (deep neural network) published in

S. Spinsante et al. (Eds.): HealthyIoT 2022, LNICST 456, pp. 170–181, 2023.
https://doi.org/10.1007/978-3-031-28663-6_13

2012 significantly improved identification accuracy (10% higher) in comparison to traditional approaches on ImageNet's 1000 class. Since then, literature has focused on both, creating networks accurate and designing efficient in terms of computational cost. However, there is a lot of literature that discuss new architectures in terms of layer composition performance. There are few papers [1] which evaluate factors related to computational cost like execution time, memory usage, etc., and more relevantly, how computational efficiency impacts precision.

In this paper, we conduct different experiments to assess the benefits and drawbacks of the application of several existing deep neural networks (DNNs) on human activity classification. In particular, we consider the selection of 6 DNNs originally developed for image recognition and we evaluate their performance on images derived from the raw signal of an automotive FMCW Radar and then processed to obtain range-Doppler images as final output. Classification results are obtained considering the dataset in [5], made up of 171 images associated to three different activities, i.e., fast walk, slow walk and slow walk with hands in pockets. Two of these activities are very similar, so they are sometimes merged in order to achieve better results in terms of accuracy and loss functions. The dataset has been created with participants with different characteristics, such as age, sex, height and weight. Subjects walked back and forth the Radar used in the experiments within a distance of 12 m. Similar comparative studies have been developed in [2,13] on a very large dataset of plant diseases, while we test DNNs for human activity classification, which involves the resolution of different issues, starting from the small dimension of our dataset.

The rest of the paper is organized as follows. In Sect. 2 hardware and software used in our experiments are detailed. In Sect. 3 are introduced the DNN architectures. The performance metrics and the described results are finally presented in Sect. 4. Final considerations and remarks are provided in Sect. 5.

2   Materials and Methods

2.1   FMCW Radar

Frequency Modulated Continuous Wave (FMCW) Radar technology has recently improved its presence on the market due to its growing application in the automotive field. Devices that apply this technology are able to detect targets and to measure their velocity and angle of arrival. A simplified block scheme of this type of sensors is depicted in Fig. 1.

Angular information can be obtained with a Multiple-In-Multiple-Out (MIMO) sensor. In communications MIMO is generally used to improve the data throughput, while in Radar systems this technology is used to obtain the angle information exploiting the different phases of the echoed signals [6,11,19]. Thanks to the characteristics of radar sensors working with carrier frequencies between 77 to 81 [GHz] and given the wavelength involved, it is possible to obtain very interesting and precise information about the targets. In particular, the micro-Doppler extracted from the processing of these types of Radar signals can be exploited for classification purposes [14,16].

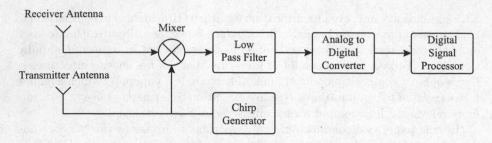

Fig. 1. FMCW Radar block scheme.

The dataset considered in the present work consists of range-Doppler maps, each of these images containing the micro-Doppler information related to different activities. The data processing necessary to obtain the maps from raw data is as follows. The considered sensor is the AWR1642, which is connected to the DCA1000 FPGA. A second board is used to configure the Radar sensor, collect the data, and stream the raw samples on the computer [8,9]. AWR1642 uses two-transmitter and four-receiver MIMO antennas. This means that the analog-to-digital converters sample four beat signals, which are then summed together. The summation improves the signal-to-noise ratio of the maps. At this point, only one signal is obtained and it is then reorganized into a Fast-Time/Slow-Time matrix. The Fast-Time represents the sample collection time (i.e., the sampling time of the analog-to-digital converters), while the Slow-Time represents the pulse repetition interval. An example of this map is reported in Fig. 2.

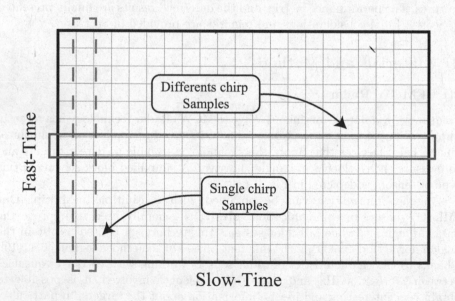

Fig. 2. Example of Fast-Time/Slow-Time matrix.

From these data matrices, it is possible to obtain the range-Doppler maps by performing a Fast Fourier Transform (FFT) along the Fast-Time axis and along the Slow-Time axis. The range-Doppler maps can be therefore used to train and test the classification algorithms. An example of the result of the whole pre-processing operation is shown in Fig. 3.

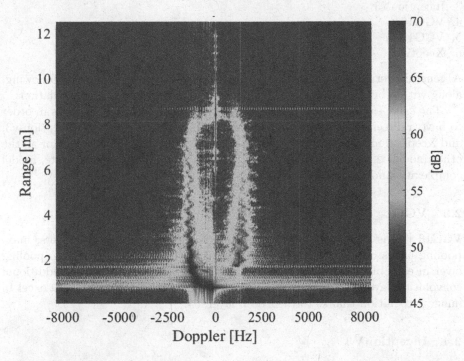

Fig. 3. Example of Range-Doppler map. Fast-Time has been converted into range distance and Slow-Time into Doppler.

2.2   Overview of CNNs

In this section, we provide a brief description of the CNNs architectures considered for our experiments. Because of the small dimension of the dataset in [5], transfer learning is applied [17]. TensorFlow package 2.3.0 is used to process neural networks with CUDA-V11.0 and cuDNN-v7.1 as the back-end.

A CNN architecture is made up of different layers, namely, the convolutional layer, pooling layer, reLU layer, fully connected layer, and loss layer. The convolutional layer is the main component of a CNN, comprising of filters (or *kernels*) that identify and forward various sorts of characteristics from the input. A pooling layer is included between consecutive convolutional layers to minimize the parameters in the network. The ReLu layer is a function that converts the negative numbers to zero.

We choose several types of networks, some of which are meant to be even more effective in terms of performance related to our small dataset. In certain situations, the number that appears with the name of architecture represents the number of layers containing parameters to be learned (e.g., convolutional, or fully connected layers). The considered architectures are the following:

1. ResNet50
2. Inception ResNetV2
3. InceptionV3
4. VGG16
5. VGG19
6. Xception

A general overview of the different architectures is provided in the following, along with a brief description of the optimizers considered in our simulations.

The same sampling policies are applied to all the selected networks in order to have a direct fair and precise comparison. InceptionResNet-v2, Inception-v3, and Xception models require normalized images with 229 pixels, while for all the other models 224 pixels are used. Our study is focused on accuracy rate, model complexity, and inference time.

2.3   VGG

VGG16 [18] is composed by 16 levels divided into convolutional layers, max-pooling layers, and fully linked layers. It has 5 blocks and a maximum pooling layer in each block. Similarly, VGG19 contains 19 layers, with three additional convolution layers in the last three blocks. Both VGG16 and VGG19 excel in image recognition thanks to their deep layers.

2.4   InceptionV3

Deep convolutional architecture Inception V3 is frequently used for classification problems. Szegedy et al. [20] first suggested the model notion in the Google Net architecture where this model is proposed by upgrading the inception module. Each block of the Inception V3 network contains many branches of convolutions, average pooling, max pooling, concatenated, dropouts, and fully connected layers, with each block having several symmetric and symmetric construction blocks. The network contains 42 layers and 29.3 million parameters; thus, its computing cost is only around 2.5 times that of GoogleNet. The combination of a reduced parameter count and additional regularization with batch-normalized auxiliary classifiers and label-smoothing allows for training higher quality networks on small training sets.

2.5   Residual Network (ResNet)

He et al. [7] developed the ResNet models, which are based on deep architectures that have demonstrated strong convergence tendencies and convincing correctness. ResNet was created using many stacked residual units and a variety of layers. However, depending on the design, the number of operations can be changed.

Convolutional, pooling, and layers make up the residual units for all the above. ResNet is comparable to VGG net but it is eight times deeper. The ResNet 50 network has 49 convolutional layers and a fully linked layer at the end.

2.6 Xception

Xception [3] is based on depthwise separable convolutional layers. This neural network architecture has 36 convolutional layers. In this way, the feature extraction base of the network is formed. Except for the first and the last modules, all thirty six layers are divided into 14 modules, all of which contain linear residual connections surrounding them. In summary, the Xception design is a depthwise separable convolution layer stack with residual connections. This lets the architecture be easily modifiable and defined simply using high-level libraries.

2.7 Optimizers

Gradient descent is the most used method to improve the learning of deep neural networks. It basically updates each model parameter, verifying how it affects the objective function, and iterates until this function converges to the minimum. Stochastic Gradient Descent (SGD) is a well known variation of gradient descent. The Adaptive Gradient Algorithm (Adagrad) optimizer [4] is designed to deal with sparse data. It adapts the learning rate to the parameters, performing smaller updates (i.e. low learning rates) for parameters associated with frequently occurring features, and larger updates (i.e. high learning rates) for parameters associated with infrequent features. Adadelta is instead an extension of Adagrad developed in [24], simultaneously to Root Mean Square Propagation (RMSprop), with the aim of solving Adagrad's diminishing learning rates. Adaptive Moment Estimation (Adam) [10] is another method that computes adaptive learning rates for each parameter.

3 Proposed Methodology

As already mentioned in the previous sections, the dataset in [5] is considered. Dataset was built at Marche Polytechnic University. Different subjects of age, sex, height, and weight participate in the tests, repeating each activity (slow walk, fast walk and walk with the hands in pockets) three times. A total of 171 images of 224×224 pixels are built. The raw data obtained from the Radar are processed to obtain range-Doppler maps as described in Sect. 2.1 and feature detection is applied to smooth the signals.

The proposed methodology is conceptualized in Fig. 4. All the images are colored (RGB). Classification is performed by exploiting the range-Doppler maps. Data Augmentation is used to pre-process the range-Doppler images to remove noise or redundancy. Also, it increases accuracy and rushes the execution. For this purpose, Keras deep learning library in Python is used. When a large amount

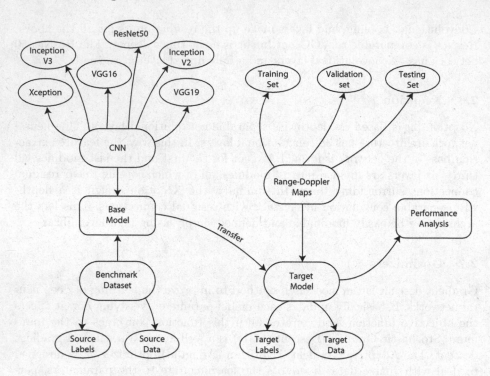

Fig. 4. Conceptual model of the proposed methodology.

of data is available, a model is built from scratch to solve a specific problem. Differently, when the dataset dimension is small, transfer learning is usually applied, and a model built by training on a larger dataset can be used as a starting point to train the network on our specific data.

Numerous pre-trained models are available under certain conditions. For our implementation, we used six pre-trained models, namely, VGG16, VGG19, InceptionResNetV2, InceptionV3, ResNet50, Xception. We fine-tuned all the models on the last layer. All 171 images are randomly generated using ImageDataGenerator. Training and testing image datasets used the same data generators. These ImageDataGenerators apply pre-processing while generating the images. We also use label encoding to get the categorical output. When the validation accuracy stops improving, early stopping is used to terminate the training process. The underlying model is then combined by a GlobalAveragePooling layer, which is used to reduce the data and prepare the model for the final classification. After that, a BatchNormalization layer is introduced for model stability and to have a faster execution, resulting in fewer training epochs. The last layer exploits a dense layer and a SoftMax activation function for extracting and categorizing the output. The weights are updated using different optimizers with an activation function of softmax in the final layer for classifying output. Optimizers are used to update the weights. The performance of the network is measured using a categorical loss function. A dropout is added to avoid overfitting.

After verifying that a number greater than 100 epochs leads to overfitting, the models are trained using a size batch of 50 and 100 epochs on the training set and then tested on the test set. At the end we evaluate the performance of the chosen models as a function of different parameters.

4   Experiments and Results

We here present a comparison of the results obtained by applying different neural networks and different optimizers to the dataset in [5]. For the sake of reproducibility, we select a random seed equal to 1337. This choice does not influence the results, since they are averaged over multiple random selections. The dataset then is randomly split into 80% for training, 10% for validation, and 10% for testing. This is done to prevent results from repeating each time the algorithm is rerun. The considered output classes are:

- Fast walk;
- Slow walk;
- Slow walk with hands into pockets.

We first define the metrics which will be used to evaluate the performance of the proposed methodologies. They are based on the so-called *confusion matrix*, whose columns represent the predicted values for each class, while the rows represent the real values. The most common metric is the accuracy, which is defined as

$$Acc = \frac{TP + TN}{TP + TN + FP + FN},\tag{1}$$

where TP and TN stand for true positives and true negatives, while FP and FN are the false positives and the false negatives.

A loss function measures the probabilities or uncertainty of a prediction based on how much the prediction varies from the true value. Differently from accuracy, the loss is computed as a summation of the errors made for each sample in training or validation sets, and is not evaluated as a percentage. Loss is often used in the training process to find the "best" parameter values for the model (e.g. weights in neural network). During the training process, the goal is to minimize this value. In the following, we consider the categorical cross-entropy loss.

Another useful metric is the precision (also called positive predictive value), which corresponds to the ratio of correctly predicted positive observations to the total predicted positive observations or

$$P = TP/(TP + FP).\tag{2}$$

Recall (also known as sensitivity) is the ratio of correctly predicted positive observations to all observations in actual class

$$R = TP/(TP + FN).\tag{3}$$

Table 1. Accuracy and loss for two activities. Accuracy values are reported as percentages.

Model	VGG16		ResNet50		Inception ResNetV2		InceptionV3		Xception		VGG19	
Optimizer	ACC	LOSS	ACC	LOSS	ACC	LOSS	ACC	LOSS	ACC	LOSS	ACC	LOSS
Adam	93.75	0.17	85.71	0.32	95.92	0.63	97.96	0.11	93.97	0.13	93.75	0.29
RMSprop	93.75	0.17	81.63	0.36	97.96	0.06	97.96	0.05	97.96	0.07	93.75	0.25
SGD	87.50	0.27	67.35	0.54	89.80	0.22	95.92	0.16	91.84	0.20	81.25	0.37
Adadelta	81.25	0.48	67.35	0.51	89.80	0.27	87.76	0.25	89.80	0.25	81.25	0.50
Adagrad	93.75	0.19	89.80	0.34	97.96	0.04	95.92	0.06	97.96	0.06	93.75	0.27
Adamax	93.75	0.17	89.80	0.40	97.96	0.07	97.96	0.05	95.92	0.14	93.75	0.29

Table 2. Accuracy and loss for three activities. Accuracy values are reported as percentages.

Model	VGG16		ResNet50		Inception ResNetV2		InceptionV3		Xception		VGG19	
Optimizer	ACC	LOSS	ACC	LOSS	ACC	LOSS	ACC	LOSS	ACC	LOSS	ACC	LOSS
Adam	60	0.66	53.3	0.74	66.7	2.2	66.7	0.51	66.67	3.44	66.67	0.75
RMSprop	66.7	0.74	53.3	0.91	80	1.1	86.7	1.49	80	1.70	73.3	0.68
SGD	60	0.94	33.3	1.08	73.3	0.66	86.7	0.56	60	0.85	53.3	0.89
Adadelta	60	1.01	53.3	0.99	53.3	0.77	60	0.65	60	0.77	60	0.97
Adagrad	53.3	0.68	60	0.82	80	0.77	66.7	0.66	73.3	0.87	53.3	0.74
Adamax	80	0.67	46.6	0.82	80	0.90	86.7	2.50	66.7	1.30	60	0.77

The F1 score is the harmonic mean of the precision and recall, where an F1 score reaches its best value at 1 (perfect precision and recall). Therefore, this score takes both false positives and false negatives into account as follows

$$F1 = 2RP/(R + P). \qquad (4)$$

The accuracy and loss for two and three activities are shown in Tables 1 and 2, respectively. Different optimizers are selected for each type of CNN. In the two-activities test, we have an imbalance between the folders because the slow walk and slow walk with hands in pockets classes are merged. This gives us some fluctuation in the results of the training and validation loss. It is possible to rve that the Inception family of algorithms leads to the best results for the two activities case, especially when the RMSprop optimizer is selected. The small dimension of the dataset deeply affects the results when three different activities are considered, as evident from the high values of the loss function. This reflects the fact that there are not enough images to perform a correct classification, and the model easily tends to overfit. An accuracy of more than 86% is however achieved by InceptionV3 network is SGD optimizer, with an overall contained loss with respect to the other cases.

In Table 3 we report the precision and recall values and the F1 score for three CNNs, i.e., VGG16, ResNet50 and Inception ResNetV2. We select the optimizers which give the best results and corresponds to Adagrad, RMSprop and Adam, respectively. In general, there is no CNN or optimizers which results the best in all cases, so a suitable configuration must be selected depending on the scenario and the parameters that we want to maximize.

Table 3. Precision, recall and F1 score for the FastWalk and SlowWalk activities.

Model	VGG16			ResNet50			Inception ResNetV2		
	P	R	F1	P	R	F1	P	R	F1
FastWalk	1	0.43	0.6	1	0.57	0.73	0.6	0.43	0.5
SlowWalk	0.75	1	0.86	0.8	1	0.89	0.71	0.83	0.77

Table 4. Execution times required by different algorithms for the three activities case. All times are reported in seconds.

Model	VGG16	ResNet50	Inception ResNetV2	InceptionV3	Xception	VGG19
Adam	30	100	38	55	107	21.04
RMSprop	52	195	75	93	150	42.4
SGD	19	68	24	30	47	17

Finally, in Tables 4 and 5 we compare the execution times required by each algorithm. Indeed, complexity and duration of running algorithms is an important parameter to take into account when dealing with IoT devices, which have limited storage and computational capacity. Algorithms have been tested using a Windows 10 Pro 64-bit (10.0, Build19042.789), Version 20H2, Intel Core I7-5500U, CPU @ 2.40 Ghz RAM 16 GB, Display NVIDIA GeForce 920M 4 GB. In this case there are no evident differences between the cases with two or three activities. In both scenarios SGD takes less time than other optimizers, while VGG19 results the fastest network. SGD in fact is a variation of the classical gradient descent, but it only computes a tiny subset or random selection of data instances, rather than the entire dataset, which is redundant and wasteful. In this way SGD needs less iterations until the objective function converges to the minimum, thus resulting faster than other optimizers, and when the learning rate is modest, it is able to achieve the same results than traditional gradient descent. Adam is instead a gradient-based optimization technique for stochastic objective functions. It computes specific adaptive learning rates for distinct parameters by combining the benefits of two SGD extensions, RMSProp and AdaGrad. Although it has a great popularity, Adam has recently been shown to fail to converge to an optimal solution in some situations, thus requiring in some cases larger execution times.

Table 5. Execution times required by different algorithms for the two activities case. All times are reported in seconds.

Model	VGG16	ResNet50	Inception ResNetV2	InceptionV3	Xception	VGG19
Adam	31.2	196	45.7	57.2	114	24
RMSprop	56.1	104	89	117	215	60
SGD	19	86	39	42.1	73	24

5   Conclusions

Deep learning is a branch of artificial intelligence that is widely applied in different fields. We have considered human activity classification performed by exploiting images derived from an automotive Radar, which represents an emerging contactless technology. We have shown how different pre-trained models built using transfer learning can achieve good results to discriminate different gait velocities. In order to define a solution which is more easily implementable on IoT devices with limited capacity, we have provided a comparison between different neural networks, in terms of accuracy, loss, classification parameters and execution times. The quality of health monitoring and the detection of smaller movements, including the position of hands during walking, can be further improved by expanding the dataset dimension and including the tracking of the subjects and trajectory.

References

1. Bianco, S., Cadene, R., Celona, L., Napoletano, P.: Benchmark analysis of representative deep neural network architectures. IEEE Access **6**, 64270–64277 (2018)
2. Chellapandi, B., Vijayalakshmi, M., Chopra, S.: Comparison of pre-trained models using transfer learning for detecting plant disease. In: 2021 International Conference on Computing, Communication, and Intelligent Systems (ICCCIS), pp. 383–387. IEEE (2021)
3. Chollet, F.: Xception: deep learning with depthwise separable convolutions. In: Proceedings of the IEEE Conference on Computer Vision and Pattern Recognition, pp. 1251–1258 (2017)
4. Duchi, J., Hazan, E., Singer, Y.: Adaptive subgradient methods for online learning and stochastic optimization. J. Mach. Learn. Res. **12**(7), 2121–2159 (2011)
5. Gambi, E., Ciattaglia, G., De Santis, A., Senigagliesi, L.: Millimeter wave radar data of people walking. Data Brief **31**, 105996 (2020). https://doi.org/10.1016/j.dib.2020.105996, https://www.sciencedirect.com/science/article/pii/S2352340920308908
6. Haimovich, A.M., Blum, R.S., Cimini, L.J.: Mimo radar with widely separated antennas. IEEE Signal Process. Mag. **25**(1), 116–129 (2007)
7. He, K., Zhang, X., Ren, S., Sun, J.: Deep residual learning for image recognition. In: Proceedings of the IEEE Conference on Computer Vision and Pattern Recognition, pp. 770–778 (2016)

8. Instruments, T.: Awr1642 single-chip 77- and 79-ghz fmcw radar sensor. http://w3techs.com/technologies/overview/contentlanguage/all

9. Instruments, T.: Dca1000evm data capture card. http://www.ti.com/lit/ug/spruij4a/spruij4a.pdf

10. Kingma, D.P., Ba, J.: Adam: A method for stochastic optimization. arXiv preprint arXiv:1412.6980 (2014)

11. Krieger, G.: Mimo-sar: opportunities and pitfalls. IEEE Trans. Geosci. Remote Sens. **52**(5), 2628–2645 (2013)

12. Krizhevsky, A., Sutskever, I., Hinton, G.E.: Imagenet classification with deep convolutional neural networks. Adv. Neural. Inf. Process. Syst. **25**, 1097–1105 (2012)

13. Maeda-Gutierrez, V., et al.: Comparison of convolutional neural network architectures for classification of tomato plant diseases. Appl. Sci. **10**(4), 1245 (2020)

14. Pan, E.: Object classification using range-doppler plots from a high density PMCW mimo mmwave radar (2020)

15. Ryu, S.J., Suh, J.S., Baek, S.H., Hong, S., Kim, J.H.: Feature-based hand gesture recognition using an FMCW radar and its temporal feature analysis. IEEE Sens. J. **18**(18), 7593–7602 (2018). https://doi.org/10.1109/JSEN.2018.2859815

16. Senigagliesi, L., Ciattaglia, G., De Santis, A., Gambi, E.: People walking classification using automotive radar. Electronics **9**(4), 588 (2020)

17. Shu, M.: Deep learning for image classification on very small datasets using transfer learning (2019)

18. Simonyan, K., Zisserman, A.: Very deep convolutional networks for large-scale image recognition. arXiv preprint arXiv:1409.1556 (2014)

19. Sun, S., Petropulu, A.P., Poor, H.V.: Mimo radar for advanced driver-assistance systems and autonomous driving: advantages and challenges. IEEE Signal Process. Mag. **37**(4), 98–117 (2020)

20. Szegedy, C., et al.: Going deeper with convolutions. In: 2015 IEEE Conference on Computer Vision and Pattern Recognition (CVPR), pp. 1–9 (2015). https://doi.org/10.1109/CVPR.2015.7298594

21. Vandersmissen, B., et al.: Indoor person identification using a low-power FMCW radar. IEEE Trans. Geosci. Remote Sens. **56**(7), 3941–3952 (2018). https://doi.org/10.1109/TGRS.2018.2816812

22. Wang, Y., Ren, A., Zhou, M., Wang, W., Yang, X.: A novel detection and recognition method for continuous hand gesture using FMCW radar. IEEE Access **8**, 167264–167275 (2020). https://doi.org/10.1109/ACCESS.2020.3023187

23. Wu, W., Dasgupta, S., Ramirez, E.E., Peterson, C., Norman, G.J.: Classification accuracies of physical activities using smartphone motion sensors. J. Med. Internet Res. **14**(5), e130 (2012)

24. Zeiler, M.D.: Adadelta: an adaptive learning rate method. arXiv preprint arXiv:1212.5701 (2012)

25. Zhang, L., Wu, X., Luo, D.: Recognizing human activities from raw accelerometer data using deep neural networks. In: 2015 IEEE 14th International Conference on Machine Learning and Applications (ICMLA), pp. 865–870. IEEE (2015)

Author Index

© ICST Institute for Computer Sciences, Social Informatics and Telecommunications Engineering 2023
Published by Springer Nature Switzerland AG 2023. All Rights Reserved
S. Spinsante et al. (Eds.): HealthyIoT 2022, LNICST 456, pp. 183–184, 2023.
https://doi.org/10.1007/978-3-031-28663-6

Printed in the United States
by Baker & Taylor Publisher Services